Information Technology

for the

Health Professions

Second Edition

Lillian Burke

Barbara Weill

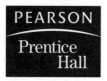

PEARSON

Prentice
Hall

Upper Saddle River, New Jersey

Library of Congress Cataloging-in-Publication Data

Burke, Lillian.
  Information technology for the health professions / Lillian Burke, Barbara Weill.
— 2nd ed.
      p. ; cm.
  Includes bibliographical references and index.
  ISBN 0-13-117592-0
  [DNLM: 1. Medical Informatics.   2. Information Systems.   W 26.5 B959i 2005]
R858.B856 2005
610'.285—dc22

                                                    2004014880

Publisher: Julie Levin Alexander
Publisher's Assistant: Regina Bruno
Senior Acquisitions Editor: Mark Cohen
Associate Editor: Melissa Kerian
Editorial Assistant: Jaquay Felix
Director of Manufacturing and Production: Bruce Johnson
Managing Editor for Production: Patrick Walsh
Production Liaison: Christina Zingone
Production Editor: Karen Berry/Pine Tree Composition, Inc.
Manufacturing Manager: Ilene Sanford
Manufacturing Buyer: Pat Brown
Creative Director: Cheryl Asherman

Senior Design Coordinator: Christopher Weigand
Cover Designer: Kevin Kall
Director of Marketing/Marketing Manager: Karen Allman
Channel Marketing Manager: Rachele Strober
Marketing Coordinator: Janet Ryerson
Media Editor: John Jordan
Media Production Manager: Amy Peltier
Media Project Manager: Stephen Hartner
Composition: Pine Tree Composition
Printer/Binder: RR Donnelley & Sons, VA
Cover Printer: Phoenix Color Corporation

We wish to thank Martin Krusin for his invaluable assistance.

Credits and acknowledgments borrowed from other sources and reproduced, with permission, in this textbook appear on appropriate page within text.

Microsoft® and Windows® are registered trademarks of the Microsoft Corporation in the U.S.A. and other countries. Screen shots and icons reprinted with permission from the Microsoft Corporation. This book is not sponsored or endorsed by or affiliated with the Microsoft Corporation.

Pearson Prentice Hall™ is a trademark of Pearson Education, Inc.
Pearson® is a registered trademark of Pearson plc
Prentice Hall® is a registered trademark of Pearson Education, Inc.

Pearson Education LTD.
Pearson Education Singapore, Pte. Ltd
Pearson Education, Canada, Ltd
Pearson Education–Japan
Pearson Education Australia PTY, Limited

Pearson Education North Asia Ltd
Pearson Educación de Mexico, S.A. de C.V.
Pearson Education Malaysia, Pte. Ltd
Pearson Education, Upper Saddle River, New Jersey

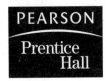

10 9 8 7 6 5 4 3 2 1
ISBN 0-13-117592-0

To our families, for their inspiration, understanding, patience, faith in us, and love.

Molly and Harry, Richard, Andrea and Daniel

—L.B.

Hazel and Rob, Mike, Buffy and Dan, Joanne and Melissa and Sarah

—B.W.

Contents

Preface xiii

Reviewers xvii

CHAPTER 1 *Introduction to Information Technology—Hardware, Software, and Telecommunications* **1**

Outline 1

Learning Objectives 2

Information Technology and Computer Literacy 2

What Is a Computer? 2

Hardware 3

    Digital and Analog Devices 3

    Input Devices 4

    Processing Hardware and Memory 5

    Open Architecture 6

    Output Devices 6

    Secondary Storage Devices 6

Software 6

    System Software 7

    Application Software 7

An Overview of Networking, Connectivity, and Telecommunications 8

    Protocols 9

Communications Hardware 9

    Analog and Digital Signals: The Modem 9

Uses of Telecommunications and Networking 9

The Internet and the World Wide Web 9

    Intranets/Extranets 10

    Internet Services 10

    The World Wide Web 10

Chapter Summary 11

Key Terms 12

Review Questions 13

   Multiple Choice 13

   True/False Questions 15

   Critical Thinking 15

Sources 16

Related Web Sites 17

CHAPTER 2 *Security and Privacy in an Electronic Age* **19**

Outline 19

Learning Objectives 20

Security and Privacy—An Overview 20

Threats to Information Technology 21

   Computer Technology and Crime 21

   Security 22

Privacy 25

Databases 26

   Government Databases 27

   Private Databases 28

   Databases and the Internet 29

Privacy, Security, and Health Care 29

   Health Insurance Portability and Accountability Act (HIPAA) of 1996 30

   Privacy of Medical Records under HIPAA and the USA Patriot Act 31

   Telemedicine and Privacy 32

   E-mail and Privacy 32

   Privacy and Electronic Medical Records 32

Chapter Summary 34

Key Terms 34

Review Questions 35

   Multiple Choice 35

   True/False Questions 37

   Critical Thinking 37

Sources 38

Related Web Site 40

CHAPTER 3 *An Introduction to Medical Informatics and the Administrative Applications of Computers* **41**

Outline 41

Learning Objectives 41

Medical Informatics 42

Administrative Applications of Computer Technology
     in the Medical Office 43

Medical Office Administrative Software—An Overview 44

The Patient Information Form 45

The Electronic Medical Record 45

Coding and Grouping 46

Accounting, Using MediSoft 46

Insurance 47

Claims 48

Accounting Reports 51

Other Systems 51

Chapter Summary 52

Key Terms 53

Review Questions 53

Definitions 53

Multiple Choice 54

True/False Questions 55

Critical Thinking 56

Sources 56

CHAPTER 4 *Telemedicine*   **59**

Outline 59

Learning Objectives 59

Overview 60

Store-and-Forward Technology and Interactive Videoconferencing 61

Teleradiology 61

Telepathology 62

Teledermatology 62

Telecardiology 63

Telestroke 63

Telepsychiatry 64

Remote Monitoring Devices 65

Telehome Care 65

Telemedicine in Prison 66

Other Uses of Telemedicine 67

The Telenurse 68

Issues in Telemedicine 68

Selected Reading 70
Chapter Summary 71
Key Terms 71
Review Questions 72
  Multiple Choice 72
  True/False Questions 74
  Critical Thinking 74
Sources 74
Related Web Sites 78

CHAPTER   5 *Information Technology in Radiology*   79

Outline 79
Learning Objectives 79
Introduction 80
X-rays 80
Ultrasound 81
Digital Imaging Techniques 82
  Computerized Tomography 82
  Magnetic Resonance Imaging 83
  Positron Emission Tomography 84
  Bone Density Tests 86
Bloodless Surgery 86
Selected Reading 87
Chapter Summary 89
Key Terms 89
Review Questions 89
  Multiple Choice 89
  True/False Questions 91
  Critical Thinking 91
Sources 91

CHAPTER   6 *Information Technology in Dentistry*   95

Outline 95
Learning Objectives 96
Overview 96
Education 96

Administrative Applications 97
   The Electronic Dental Chart 97
Demographics and the Transformation of Dentistry 100
Computerized Instruments in Dentistry 102
Endodontics 102
Periodontics 103
Cosmetic Dentistry 103
Diagnosis and Expert Systems 103
Diagnostic Tools 104
   X-rays 104
   Digital Radiography 104
   Electrical Conductance 106
   Emerging Methods 106
   Light Illumination 106
Lasers in Dentistry 106
Minimally Invasive Dentistry 108
Surgery 109
The Growth of Specialization 109
Teledentistry 109
Selected Reading 109
Chapter Summary 110
Key Terms 111
Review Questions 111
   Multiple Choice 111
   True/False Questions 112
   Critical Thinking 113
Sources 113

CHAPTER 7 *Information Technology in Surgery*   **115**

Outline 115
Learning Objectives 115
Overview 116
Computer-Assisted Surgery 116
   Computer-Assisted Surgical Planning 116
   Minimally Invasive Surgery (MIS) 117
   Computer-Assisted Surgery and Robotics 118
   ROBODOC, AESOP, ZEUS, da Vinci, MINERVA, and Other Robotic Devices 119
   Augmented Reality 122

Telepresence Surgery 123

Discussion and Future Directions 124

Lasers in Surgery 124

Conclusion 124

Selected Reading 125

Chapter Summary 126

Key Terms 127

Review Questions 127

Multiple Choice 127

True/False Questions 128

Critical Thinking 129

Sources 129

CHAPTER   8 *Information Technology in Pharmacy*   **133**

Outline 133

Learning Objectives 134

Overview 134

Biotechnology and the Human Genome Project 134

Rational Drug Design 134

Bioinformatics 135

The Human Genome Project 135

Developments in Biotechnology 136

Computer-Assisted Drug Trials 137

Computer-Assisted Drug Review 138

The Computerized Pharmacy 138

Computers and Drug Errors 138

The Automated Community Pharmacy 140

Automating the Hospital Pharmacy 142

The Hospital Pharmacy Robot and Bar Codes 142

Point-of-Use Drug Dispensing 142

Telepharmacy 143

Drug Delivery on a Chip 145

The Impact of Information Technology on Pharmacy 145

Selected Reading 146

Chapter Summary 148

Key Terms 148

Review Questions 149

Multiple Choice 149

True/False Questions 150

Critical Thinking 150

Sources 151

CHAPTER 9 *Computerized Medical Devices, Assistive Technology, and Prosthetic Devices 155*

Outline 155

Learning Objectives 155

Overview 156

Computerized Medical Instruments 156

Computerized Devices in Optometry/Opthalmology 157

Assistive Devices 158

Augmentative Communications Devices 160

Environmental Control Systems 161

Prosthetic Devices 162

CFES Technology 165

Risks Posed by Implants 166

Conclusion 166

Selected Readings 166

Chapter Summary 169

Key Terms 170

Review Questions 170

Multiple Choice 170

True/False Questions 171

Critical Thinking 172

Sources 172

CHAPTER 10 *Informational Resources: Computer-Assisted Instruction, Expert Systems, and Health Information Online 175*

Outline 175

Learning Objectives 176

Overview 176

Education 176

The Visible Human 176

Computer-Assisted Instruction 177

Simulation Software 178

Virtual Reality Simulations 178

Patient Simulators 181

Distance Learning 181

Decision Support: Expert Systems 185

Health Information on the Internet 186

Medical Literature Databases 187

E-mail 189

Self-help on the Web 192

Support Groups on the Web 193

Judging the Reliability of Health Information on the Internet 194

Self-help Software 195

Conclusion 195

Selected Reading 196

Chapter Summary 197

Key Terms 198

Review Questions 198

Multiple Choice 198

True/False Questions 199

Critical Thinking 200

Sources 200

Related Web Sites 203

CHAPTER 11 *Conclusion and Future Directions*   205

Outline 205

Learning Objectives 205

Overview 205

Clinical and Special Purpose Applications: Future Trends 206

Administrative Applications: The Integrated Electronic
Medical Record 208

Demographic Changes and Occupational Outlooks
for Health Care Professionals 210

Social Implications 211

Chapter Summary 211

Sources 212

Glossary   215

Index   229

Preface

Information technology continues to change many aspects of society, including health care and its delivery. In *Information Technology for the Health Professions,* we take a practical approach to introducing health care professionals to the myriad uses of computer technology in health care fields. After a brief introduction to the essential concepts needed to understand computer hardware, software, telecommunications, and the privacy and security of information, we see how these technologies have affected various aspects of health care. The term information technology includes not only computers, but also communications networks and computer literacy, that is, knowledge of the uses of computer technology. Rapidly changing computer technology continues to exert a major influence on all aspects of society. The understanding of the interconnections of hardware, software, networks, and new medical techniques is essential.

AN INTRODUCTION TO THE SECOND EDITION

The second edition of *Information Technology for the Health Professions* has been expanded and updated for the new millennium. It includes new sections on recent technological developments and their uses in health care and its delivery, on new laws affecting privacy and security of medical information, an expanded chapter on medical informatics and the administrative uses of computers, and a new chapter on computer technology in dentistry. Dated materials have been deleted. Although *Information Technology* is geared to an audience interested in health care, it is written at a level appropriate for the layperson.

Chapter 1: Introduction to Information Technology— Hardware, Software, and Telecommunications

The first three chapters of the first edition on computer literacy, computer hardware and software, and networking and telecommunications have been condensed, keeping only information essential to students and others interested in computers and health care. These chapters have been combined into a new Chapter 1, which provides the student with information necessary to anyone living and working in a computerized society.

Chapter 2: Security and Privacy in an Electronic Age

Chapter 2 deals with the problems of security and privacy of information in electronic form and on networks. Both general issues of security and privacy in an electronic age and problems specific to health care are discussed. New issues of security and privacy are raised by new laws. The student is introduced to the Health Information Portability and Accountability Act of 1996 (HIPAA) that provides the first national minimum standards for the privacy of medical information. The book also deals with the effects of the USA Patriot Act on medical privacy.

Chapter 3: An Introduction to Medical Informatics and the Administrative Applications of Computers

Chapter 3 is an expanded introduction to medical informatics—the use of technology to organize information in health care. The student is introduced to the traditional classifications of clinical uses of computers (used in direct patient care); administrative uses of computers used in office administration, financial planning, billing, and scheduling; and the special purpose uses of computers in education and pharmacy. The chapter has an expanded section on the administrative uses of computers discussing the computerization of tasks in the medical office, the electronic medical record, and bucket billing. It also introduces the student to grouping and coding systems, insurance, and the various accounting reports used in the health care environment.

Chapter 4: Telemedicine

Chapter 4 deals with telemedicine and its rapid expansion. Telecommunications and connectivity have made possible telemedicine, from the simple sharing of patient records or X-rays over networks, to distance exams, to remote operation of medical instruments, to teleconferencing. The earliest telemedicine used store-and-forward technology to send images. This is still used in teleradiology, telepathology, teledermatology, telestroke programs, and telecardiology programs. Interactive videoconferencing allows a medical exam in real time—with all participants seeing and hearing each other.

Chapter 5: Information Technology in Radiology

Chapter 5 introduces the student to digital imaging techniques. Digital images (CT scans, MRIs, PET scans) are more precise than the traditional X-ray. The CT (computerized tomography) scan and MRI (magnetic resonance imaging) have become standard diagnostic tools. PET scans (positron emission tomography) allow the physician to examine the electrical and chemical processes in the brain. Currently interventional radiologists treat diseases that once required traditional surgery.

Chapter 6: Information Technology in Dentistry

A new chapter that surveys computer technology in dentistry has been added. Dentistry is changing due to changing demographics and the introduction of new computer-based techniques. During the second half of the twentieth century, dental care allowed most children to grow up with healthy teeth. Now good dental care prevents cavities in children who can afford it. An aging population seeks dental care for many reasons, including cavities, periodontal disease, and cosmetics. The fully computerized dentist's office uses the electronic medical record to integrate all aspects of care.

Chapter 7: Information Technology in Surgery

Chapter 7 surveys the uses of computers in surgery. Computers are used in surgery from the teaching and planning stages to the actual use of robotic devices in the operating room. Computer simulations help in the training of students. Minimally invasive, endoscopic surgery makes use of robotic devices to hold the endoscope.

Chapter 8: Information Technology in Pharmacy

The use of computer technology in pharmacy has traditionally been considered a special purpose application. Today, information technology is involved with medication from its design to its administration. The development of medications for the treatment of genetically-based diseases is slowly becoming a reality because of the knowledge gained through the Human Genome Project. Supercomputers, using special software, are now being used to design new medications. Software packages allow pharmacies to print out extensive drug descriptions along with side effects and interaction warnings that accompany prescription medications. Computerized infusion pumps automatically administer medication. The networking of medical devices allows a monitoring device to communicate with a drug delivery device. Robots are being used to fill prescriptions and count out capsules and tablets. Telepharmacy is expanding due to a shortage of pharmacists, a drive to cut costs, and the interest of the U.S. Department of Defense, Veterans Administration, and Immigration and Naturalization Service.

Chapter 9: Computerized Medical Devices, Assistive Technology, and Prosthetic Devices

Computer controlled medical devices include the most established clinical use of computers—the use of computerized monitoring devices. For people with disabilities, adaptive technology can make an independent life a reality. Electronic prosthetics refer to computerized replacement body parts. An artificial limb designed with the help of a computer with embedded microprocessor chips can sense and react to nerve signals. It can work like a natural limb so that a person with an electronic prosthetic foot can even participate in college sports. Some devices, such as pacemakers, make use of the technology called functional electrical stimulation, which delivers low-level electrical stimulation to muscles.

Chapter 10: Informational Resources: Computer-Assisted Instruction, Expert Systems, and Health Information Online

Computer-assisted instruction, both drill-and-practice and simulation, has long been used to educate patients and practitioners. Currently programs make use of virtual reality techniques, so the student actually feels the experience of performing a medical procedure. Online medical literature databases aid in both academic research and diagnosing patients. Expert systems try to make a computer an "expert" in one field. Interactive self-help applications include both self-help software and the use of the Internet for medical advice. Advice and information on every aspect of health care, every drug, and every disease is on the Internet.

Chapter 11: Conclusion and Future Directions

Computer technology is continuing to have an enormous impact on health care fields. Today, medical technology is in a constant state of flux. Whole new fields, such as telemedicine, are emerging and changing the way medicine is practiced. The future may hold unbelievable techniques and devices. Electronic brain implants are in their infancy, holding the promise of communication for locked-in patients as well as the threat of mind control. Other devices are currently in the testing stages. Not only are sensors being developed to help paralyzed patients move. In the future, nanotechnology may diagnose and treat disease at the molecular level.

Reviewers

Patt Elison-Bowers
Associate Professor
Health Studies
Boise State University
Boise, ID

Diane Premeau
Program Director, Health Information
    Programs
Chabot College
Hayward, CA

Pat Shaw, M.Ed, RHIA
Associate Professor
Weber State University
Ogden, UT

Philip Vuchetich
Creighton University
Omaha, NE

Deborah Weaver, RN, PhD.
Associate Professor
Valdosta State University
Valdosta, GA

Introduction to Information Technology—Hardware, Software, and Telecommunications

OUTLINE

- **Learning Objectives**
- **Information Technology and Computer Literacy**
- **What Is a Computer?**
- **Hardware**
  - *Digital and Analog Devices*
  - *Input Devices*
  - *Processing Hardware and Memory*
  - *Open Architecture*
  - *Output Devices*
  - *Secondary Storage Devices*
- **Software**
  - *System Software*
  - *Application Software*
- **An Overview of Networking, Connectivity, and Telecommunications**
  - *Protocols*
- **Communications Hardware**
  - *Analog and Digital Signals: The Modem*
- **Uses of Telecommunications and Networking**
- **The Internet and the World Wide Web**
  - *Intranets/Extranets*
  - *Internet Services*
  - *The World Wide Web*
- **Chapter Summary**
- **Key Terms**
- **Review Questions**
  - *Multiple Choice*
  - *True/False Questions*
  - *Critical Thinking*
- **Sources**
- **Related Web Sites**

LEARNING OBJECTIVES

Upon completion of this chapter, you will be able to

- Define information technology, computer, and computer literacy, and understand their significance and why you should be computer literate in today's society.
- Describe the classification of computers into supercomputers, mainframes, mini-computers, microcomputers, personal digital assistants, and embedded computers.
- Discuss the difference between digital and analog devices.
- Describe how all data and information are represented inside the computer.
- Differentiate between hardware and software and be able to discuss the different hardware components of a computer.
- Describe the difference between system and application software, know what an operating system is, and know what various application programs are used for what tasks.
- Discuss the significance of connectivity and networking.
- Identify communications media.
- List the components necessary for telecommunications to take place.
- State the uses of telecommunications and networking.

INFORMATION TECHNOLOGY AND COMPUTER LITERACY

The term **information technology (IT)** includes not only the use of computers, but also communications **networks** and **computer literacy**, that is, knowledge of how to use computer technology. As a future health care professional, familiarity with information technology is crucial. As in other fields, the basic tasks of gathering, allocating, controlling, and retrieving information are the same. In this chapter, we focus on computer literacy, computers, and networks. Currently, computer literacy involves several aspects. A computer literate person knows how to use a computer in his or her own field to make tasks easier and to complete them more efficiently, has a working knowledge of terminology, and understands in a broad general fashion what a computer is and its capabilities. Today, unlike several years ago, computer literacy involves knowledge of the **Internet** and the **World Wide Web** and the ability to take advantage of their resources.

WHAT IS A COMPUTER?

A **computer** is an electronic device that can accept **data** (raw facts) as input, process or alter them in some way, and produce useful **information** as output. A computer manipulates data by following step-by-step instructions called a **program**. The program, the data, and the information can be stored temporarily in memory while processing is going on, and then permanently on secondary storage media for future use. Computers are accurate, fast, and reliable.

HARDWARE

To understand the myriad uses of information technology in health care, you need to familiarize yourself with computer terminology, hardware, and software applications. Every computer performs similar functions.

Each function that the computer performs has **hardware** associated with it: **Input devices** take data that humans understand and input it into the computer in the digital form of offs and ons (zeroes and ones) that the computer can process; a **processing unit** manipulates data; **output devices** produce useful information for human beings; memory and **secondary storage devices** hold information, data, and programs.

Although all computers perform similar functions, all computers are not the same. There are several categories based on size, speed, and processing power. Supercomputers are the largest and most powerful computers. They are used for scientific purposes, such as weather forecasting and drug design. Mainframes are less powerful, and are used in business for input/output intensive purposes, such as generating paychecks or processing medical insurance claims. Minicomputers are scaled-down mainframes, which may be used by smaller businesses. In many environments, minicomputers have been replaced by microcomputers and networks. Microcomputers (personal computers) are powerful enough for an individual's needs in word processing, spreadsheets, and database management. Small handheld computers (personal digital assistants or PDAs) originally could hold a notepad, calendar, and an address book. Today sophisticated PDAs are used throughout the health care world. Physicians can write prescriptions, consult online databases, and capture patient information to be sent to the hospital's database using a PDA and appropriate software. The embedded computer is a single-purpose computer on a **chip** of silicon, which is embedded in anything from appliances to humans. An embedded computer may help run your car, microwave, pacemaker, or watch. A chip embedded in a human being can dispense medication among other things.

Inside the computer, whatever its size and power, data and information have to be represented in some way. In a digital computer, all information, including text, music, animation, graphics, smell, and sound, is represented by combinations of ons and offs—1s and 0s, **binary digits (bits)**. To **digitize** is to translate data into the 1s and 0s that the computer can process.

Digital and Analog Devices

The computer with which you are familiar is called a **digital device**. A digital device is one that computes by counting discrete, separate items. On the other hand, devices that aid in calculation by measuring some continuous physical property or quantity are called **analog devices**. You are familiar with both. A digital clock counts hours, minutes, and seconds. A face clock is an analog device; the distance around the clock is like (analogous to) a number of hours and minutes. A digital thermometer counts degrees of temperature. A mercury thermometer is an analog device; the length of the column of mercury is measured and is like a certain number of degrees of temperature. Both digital and analog computing devices have been developed and continue to exist, but digital computers make up the vast majority of computers. One of the areas where analog computers continue to be used is within medicine, where they may be employed to analyze blood.

The physical components of a computer are called **hardware**. Pieces of hardware can be categorized according to the functions each performs: input, process, output, storage.

Input Devices

Input devices function to take data that people understand and translate it into a form that the computer can process—that is, ons and offs. Input devices can be divided into two categories—**keyboards** and direct-entry devices.

Direct-entry devices include pointing devices, scanning devices, smart and optical cards, speech and vision input, touch screens, sensors, and human-biology input devices.

The pointing device with which you are most familiar is the **mouse**, which you can use to position the **insertion point** on the screen, or make a choice from a menu. Other pointing devices are variations of the mouse and include the trackpad (used with laptops) and the joystick (used with games). Light pens, digitizing tablets, and pen-based systems allow you to use a pen or stylus to enter data. The marks you make or letters you write are digitized so that the computer can process them.

Most **scanning devices** digitize data by shining a light on an image and measuring the reflection. Bar-code scanners read the universal product codes on products, optical mark recognition (OMR) can recognize a mark on paper, and optical character recognition (OCR) devices can recognize letters. Special scanning equipment called magnetic ink character recognition (MICR) is used by banks to read the numbers at the bottoms of checks. You are familiar with fax machines, which scan images, digitize them, and send them over phone wires. Some scanning devices, called image scanners, can scan and digitize whole pages of text and graphics. One scanning device of particular interest to those with impaired eyesight is the Kurzweil scanner, which scans printed text and reads it aloud to the user.

Several different kinds of cards are used as input devices. Your ATM card or charge card contains a small amount of data in the magnetic stripe. A smart card can hold more data, and contains a microprocessor. Smart cards have been used as debit cards. Several states now use smart cards as driver's licenses. The card includes a biometric identifier, and may include other personal information as well. Privacy advocates fear that "the density of information on the cards makes them a target . . . for people trying to steal data" (Divis, 2002). The Driver's License Modernization Act of 2002 was introduced in Congress in May 2002. It would mandate that all licenses include a computer chip with a unique identifier. An optical card holds about 2,000 pages; it could be used to hold your whole medical history, including test results and X-rays. Small enough to carry in your wallet, the information on the card would be immediately available if you were hospitalized because of an emergency.

Vision input systems are currently being developed. A computer uses a digital camera to digitize images and stores the images. The computer "sees" by having the camera take a picture of an object. The digitized image of this object is then compared with the images in storage. This technology will also be used in adaptive devices, such as glasses that can help Alzheimer's patients. The glasses will include a database of names and faces; a camera sees a face, and if it "recognizes" it, the wearer is given the name of the subject.

Ideally, speech input systems allow you to talk to your computer, and the computer will be able to process the words as data and commands. A speech recognition system contains a dictionary of digital patterns of words. You say a word, and the word is then digitized and compared to the words in its dictionary. If it recognizes the word, the command is executed. There are speech dictation packages tailored to specific professions. A system geared to medicine would include an extensive vocabulary of digitized medical terms and would allow the creation of patient records and medical reports. It can be used as an input device by physicians, to dictate notes, for example, even while operating. Speech recognition is also especially beneficial as an enabling device, allowing those who do not have the use of their hands to use computers. However, speech recognition will never be perfect, simply because many phrases and words sound exactly the same, for example, hyphenate and - 8 (hyphen eight). The most up-to-date speech-recognition software allows voice correction of mistakes such as these.

Of particular interest to health professionals are input devices called sensors. A sensor is a device that collects data directly from the environment and sends it to a computer. Sensors are used to collect patient information for clinical monitoring systems, including physiological, arrhythmia, pulmonary, and obstetrical/neonatal systems. In critical care units, monitoring systems make nurses aware of any change in a patient's condition immediately. They can detect the smallest change in temperature, blood pressure, respiration, or any other physiological measurement.

The newest kind of input devices are called **human-biology input devices**. They allow you to use your body as an input device. These include **biometrics**, which are being used in security systems to protect data from unauthorized users. Biometrics identifies people by their body parts, including fingerprints, hand prints, face recognition, and iris scans. Once thought to be almost 100 percent accurate, biometric identification systems are now recognized as far from perfect. Line-of-sight input allows the user to look at a keyboard displayed on a screen, and indicate the character selected by looking at it for a prescribed amount of time. Implanted chips have allowed locked-in stroke patients to communicate with a computer by focusing brain waves (brain wave input). This is experimental and research is continuing.

Processing Hardware and Memory

Once data is inside the computer, it is processed. Processing hardware is the brain of the computer. Located on the **motherboard** (the **system board**) the **processor** or **system unit** contains the **central processing unit (CPU)** and **memory**. In a microcomputer, it is a microprocessor on a chip. In a larger computer, the processor might be on several circuit boards. The CPU has two parts: the **arithmetic-logic unit**, which performs the arithmetic operations of adding, subtracting, multiplying, dividing, and raising to a power, and the logical operation of comparing. The **control unit** directs the operation of the computer in accordance with the program's instructions.

The CPU works closely with memory. The instructions of the program being executed must be in memory for processing to take place. Memory is also located on chips on the system board. The part of memory where current work is temporarily stored during processing is called **random access memory (RAM)**. RAM is also on chips. It is temporary, volatile memory. The other part of memory (also on chips) is called **read only memory (ROM)** or firmware; it contains basic start-up instructions, which are burned into a chip at the factory. You cannot change the contents of ROM.

Open Architecture

Computers with **open architecture** allow you to add devices. The system board contains **expansion slots** into which you can plug **expansion boards** for additional hardware. The board has a socket on the outside called a **port**. You can plug a cable from your new device into the port. The significance of open architecture is the fact that it enables you to add any hardware to your existing computer system. This means not only can you expand the memory of your computer, but also you can add devices that make your computer more amenable to uses in medicine. Today medical schools use personal computers (PCs) with expansion boards to enhance their sound, video, and animation capabilities, showing interactive multimedia presentations. Expansion boards also allow the use of virtual reality simulators, which help in the teaching of certain procedures.

Output Devices

Once data is processed, output devices translate the machine language of bits into a form that humans can understand. Output devices are divided into two basic categories: those that produce **hard copy**, including **printers** and **plotters**, and those that produce **soft copy**, including **monitors** (the most commonly used output device). Soft copy is also produced by devices that produce speech, sound, or music.

Secondary Storage Devices

The memory we have discussed so far is temporary or volatile. In order to save your work more permanently, you need secondary storage devices. **Magnetic disk, magnetic tape,** and **optical disks** are used as secondary storage media. Magnetic media (disk, diskette, tape, and high-capacity Zip disks) store data and programs as magnetic spots or electromagnetic charges. High-capacity optical disks (**CDs—compact disks** or **DVDs— digital video disks**) store data as pits and lands burnt into a plastic disk by a laser.

SOFTWARE

Software refers to the programs—the step-by-step instructions that tell the hardware what to do. Without software, hardware is useless. Software falls into two general categories: **system software** and **application software**.

System Software

System software consists of programs that let the computer manage its own resources. The most important piece of system software is the **operating system.** The operating system is a group of programs that manages and organizes the resources of the computer. It controls the hardware, manages basic input and output operations, keeps track of your files saved on disk and in memory, and directs communication between the CPU and other pieces of hardware. It coordinates how other programs work with the hardware and with each other. Operating systems also provide the **user interface**, that is, the way the user communicates with the computer. For example, Windows (a widely used operating system) provides a **graphical user interface**, pictures or icons that you click on with a mouse. When the computer is turned on, the operating system is **booted** or loaded into the computer's RAM. No other program can work until the operating system is booted.

Application Software

Application software allows you to apply computer technology to a task you need done. There are application packages for many needs.

Word processing software allows you to enter text for a paper, report, letter, or memo. Once it is entered, you can format it, that is, make it look the way you want it to look. You can change the size, style, and face of the type. In addition, margins and justification can be set to any specifications. Style checkers can help you with spelling and grammar. Word processing software also includes thesauri, headers and footers, index generators, and outlining features, to name a few.

Electronic spreadsheets allow you to process numerical data. Organized into rows and columns intersecting to form cells, spreadsheets make doing arithmetic almost fun. You enter the values you want processed, the formula that tells the software how to process them, and the answer appears. If you found you made a mistake entering a value, just change it, and the answer is **automatically recalculated**. Spreadsheet software also allows you to create graphs easily just by indicating what cells you want graphed.

Database management systems permit you to manage large quantities of data in an organized fashion. Information in a database is organized in tables. The database management system makes it easy to enter data, edit it, sort or organize it, search for data that meets a particular criterion, and retrieve it. Once the structure of the table is defined and the data entered, it never has to be typed again; eye-pleasing, businesslike reports can be generated easily by simply defining their structure—not by retyping the data.

With **graphics software,** you can create all kinds of images—from simple line graphs to business presentations.

There are also specialized software packages used in such specific fields as medicine. For example, **MediSoft** is a specialized accounting program used in medical offices. Given the right software package, your computer can perform a wide variety of tasks. Computers are even being used in place of human taste-testers!

Communications software includes Web browsers, such as Netscape Navigator and Internet Explorer. These programs allow you to connect your computer to other computers in a network and to communicate via **e-mail** (electronic mail). E-mail has become a common means of communication in many businesses. However, privacy issues have prevented its widespread use in health care environments.

AN OVERVIEW OF NETWORKING, CONNECTIVITY, AND TELECOMMUNICATIONS

Communication forms the third component of information technology. The implications of telecommunications for the medical world are more fully explored in Chapter 4, Telemedicine. Although you can enjoy the wonders of the Internet and surf the World Wide Web with very little technical knowledge, this section introduces you to some of the complexities behind networking, connectivity, telecommunications, and the Internet, and gives you a foundation for appreciating the impact of these developments on health care.

Standing alone, your computer has access only to the data and information stored on its hard drive and on the disks you insert in its disk drives. However, if you can connect your PC to other computers, you have access to the data and information on their hard drives as well. The fact that computers can be connected is **connectivity**. Connectivity greatly enhances the power of your computer, bringing immense stores of information to your fingertips, and making it possible for you to interact with people around the world. Connectivity is the prerequisite for the development of the field of telemedicine. Computers and other hardware devices that are connected form what is called a network. Networks come in all sizes, from small **local area networks (LANs)** that span one room to **wide area networks (WANs)** that may span a state, nation, or even the globe, such as the Internet and World Wide Web. Networks can be private or connected via telephone lines, making them **telecommunications networks**. Given the right mix of hardware and software, computers can be connected globally.

When computers are connected, the data and information that travels between them must follow some path. There are several communications channels—both wired and wireless. Health care telecommunications need to be fast and reliable. Twisted pair—traditional phone wire—is the slowest, least expensive medium. Coaxial cable consists of a single copper core, and transmits at a higher speed. Fiber optic cable transmits as pulses of light and is the fastest medium. Some communications take place without wires via microwaves.

Most hospital telemedicine programs lease high-speed, dedicated T1 lines. At the present time, **bluetooth** technology can be used to create small personal area networks. Bluetooth is a wireless technology that can connect digital devices from computers to medical devices to cell phones. For example, if someone is wearing a pacemaker and has a heart attack, his or her cell phone will automatically dial 911.

Protocols

Transmission is governed by sets of technical standards or rules called **protocols**. They take care of how the connection is set up between devices. Protocols also establish security procedures. You do not have to think about these factors because they are embedded in the communications software.

COMMUNICATIONS HARDWARE

Analog and Digital Signals: The Modem

We defined analog and digital computing devices. They should not be confused with **analog** and **digital signals**. An analog signal is a continuous varying wave. A digital signal is a discontinuous pulse—on or off. Traditional telephone lines carry analog waves. Digital computers process digital signals. A modem translates between the two, so that data processed on a computer can be transmitted over a phone line. Higher speed alternatives include ISDN (integrated services digital network) and DSL (digital subscriber lines), which use phone wires to transmit digitally, and cable modems. T1 lines are high-speed dedicated lines.

USES OF TELECOMMUNICATIONS AND NETWORKING

The linking of computers and communications devices via telecommunications lines into networks of all sizes has made many things possible. A complete list is beyond the scope of this text. Networking allows such things as the electronic linking of health departments in what may eventually be a national Information Network for Public Health Officials, permitting the sharing of information, which can be important in containing potential epidemics. Networking makes e-mail, voice mail, teleconferencing, telecommuting, and telemedicine possible.

THE INTERNET AND THE WORLD WIDE WEB

The **Internet** (short for *inter*connected *net*work) is a global network of networks, connecting innumerable smaller networks, computers, and users. It is run by a committee of volunteers; no one owns it. The Internet originated in 1969 as **ARPAnet**, a project of the Advanced Research Projects Agency of the U.S. Department of Defense. It was attempting to create both a national network of scientists and a communications system that could withstand nuclear attack. It was, therefore, to be decentralized, forming a communications web with no central authority. The protocol that eventually governed ARPAnet and continues to govern the Internet today is public domain software called **TCP/IP (transmission control protocol/Internet protocol).** Any computer or network that subscribes to this protocol can join the Internet. A computer can be directly connected to the Internet or subscribe to an **Internet service provider (ISP),** which provides a temporary connection.

Intranets/Extranets

Private corporate networks that use the same structure as the Internet and TCP/IP protocols are called **intranets.** Each computer in an intranet must have browser software. Software called a **firewall** is used to protect an intranet from unauthorized users. What the user sees looks like a Web page. Companies can use an intranet to distribute information to employees in an easy attractive format, for training videos, or to post job openings. If an intranet in one organization is linked to other intranets in other organizations, it becomes an **extranet.**

Internet Services

Once you are connected, what services are available? You can access reliable medical information databases, such as MEDLINE and AIDSLINE, through PubMed (http://www.ncbi.nlm.nih.gov/PubMed/). You can find support groups, as well as information on almost any disease, medication, hospital, and treatment. The information, which may or may not be accurate, can be so up-to-date that your physician may not even be aware of it. Internet support groups may help people cope with illness and isolation.

The World Wide Web

The **World Wide Web (WWW)** or Web is the part of the Internet that is most accessible and easiest to navigate. In 1990, a physicist, Tim Berners-Lee, conceived the Web as a way to link physicists around the world. What made the Web accessible to the general public was the creation of the first graphical browser by Marc Andreeson in 1993. The Web is made up of information organized as documents **(pages).** The information on the Web is stored in files called **Web sites.** To browse the Web, you need a connection to the Internet and software called a **Web browser.** Finding what you are looking for on the Web can be challenging. If you know the address **(URL** or **uniform resource locator),** you can just type it in. However, if you are just looking for information on a particular topic, you can use a program called a **search engine.**

The Internet and the Web provide an enormous amount of information—some of it reliable, some not. The lack of regulation, the freewheeling quality, is also an attraction, but may bring some negative consequences. *Any* information may find its way onto the Internet, and there are no safeguards for accuracy. How do you judge the reliability of medical information on the net? There are health Web sites that rate services; however, these rating services are not subject to regulation or quality control either. Recognizing the difficulty of sifting through the health information and advice on the Internet, in 1997, the Federal Department of Health and Human Services created **Healthfinder** (http://www.healthfinder.gov), a listing of "sites 'hand-picked' . . . by health professionals." Most of the sites it recommends are "government agencies, non-profit and professional organizations, universities, libraries," although it does list a few commercial sites. Along with a listing, Healthfinder provides the source of the information and a summary.

The lack of regulation applies not only to speech and information, but also to commerce. Web sites promote and sell worthless remedies. These sites play on fear—for example, promoting protection from SARS (Severe Acute Respiratory Syndrome) which first appeared in February 2003. Interpersonal interaction on the Web may also lend itself to a kind of fraud, stemming from the anonymous quality of communication through the medium of a keyboard and screen. You can neither see nor hear the person to whom you are writing. This means you are free to express aspects of your *self* that usually remain hidden. You may even present yourself as someone else.

CHAPTER SUMMARY

Chapter 1 introduces the reader to the concepts of information technology (IT) and computer literacy and their significance. It also deals with computer hardware and software and how they interact to accept data as input, process it, and produce information as output. Chapter 1 familiarizes you with networking and connectivity, telecommunications, the Internet, and the World Wide Web, and gives you the basic information you need for appreciating the significance of these developments in medicine.

- Information technology includes not only computers, but also communications networks and computer literacy.
- Computer literacy means knowledge of computers and their functions, which then makes one competent in using IT.
- A computer is an electronic device that can accept data as input, process it, and produce information as output following step-by-step instructions called a program.
- There are two different kinds of computing devices: digital devices, which compute by counting, and analog devices, which compute by measuring.
- Inside a digital computer, all data and information are represented by combinations of binary digits (bits).
- Physical components of a computer are called hardware.
- Input devices digitize data, so that the computer can process it.
  - Input devices include keyboards and direct-entry devices.
    - Direct-entry devices include pointing devices, scanning devices, smart cards, and optical cards, sensors, and human-biology input devices.

- The system unit includes the central processing unit (CPU), which is comprised of the arithmetic-logic unit and the control unit, and memory, which temporarily stores your current work. The CPU and memory work together following the instructions of a program to process data into information.
- Output devices (printers and monitors) present the processed information to the user.
- Secondary storage devices (drives) and media (diskettes, hard disks, optical disks, Zip disks, and magnetic tape) allow you to store information permanently.
- Software (programs) is comprised of the step-by-step instructions that tell the hardware how to process data.
- Software is classified as system software, which controls the basic operation of the hardware, and application software, which completes tasks for the user.
- When computers are connected in networks, the data that is transmitted travels over a path or medium.
- Data transmission is governed by technical standards or rules called protocols.
- To transmit data processed by a computer (digital signals) over traditional phone lines, which transmit analog signals, a modem (or other device) is necessary.
- The connection of computers and communications devices into networks makes many things possible, including telemedicine.
- The Internet is a global network of networks, which makes vast amounts of information available.
- The World Wide Web is part of the Internet, organized as documents with links to other documents.

KEY TERMS

analog devices	control unit	graphics software
analog signals	data	hard copy
application software	database management	hardware
arithmetic-logic unit	systems	Healthfinder
ARPAnet	digital devices	human-biology input
automatic recalculation	digital signals	devices
binary digits (bits)	digitize	information
biometrics	direct-entry devices	information technology
Bluetooth	DVDs (digital video	(IT)
booted	disks)	input devices
CDs (compact disks)	electronic mail (e-mail)	insertion point
central processing unit	electronic spreadsheets	Internet
(CPU)	e-mail	Internet service
chip	expansion boards	provider (ISP)
communications software	expansion slots	intranets
computer	extranets	keyboards
computer literacy	firewall	local area networks
connectivity	graphical user interface	(LANs)

magnetic disk
magnetic tape
MediSoft
memory
monitors
motherboard
mouse
networks
open architecture
operating system
optical disks
output devices
pages
plotters
port
printers

processing unit
processor
programs
protocols
random access memory
(RAM)
read only memory
(ROM)
scanning devices
search engine
secondary storage devices
soft copy
software
system board
system software
system unit

TCP/IP (transmission
control protocol/
Internet protocol)
telecommunications net-
works
uniform resource loca-
tor (URL)
user interface
Web browser
Web sites
wide area network
(WAN)
word processing
World Wide Web (Web
or WWW)

REVIEW QUESTIONS

Multiple Choice

1. A computer literate person _____.
   A. Can use a computer to perform tasks in his or her field
   B. Is generally familiar with what a computer can do
   C. Can program a computer
   D. A and B
2. Binary digits are used to represent _____ inside the computer.
   A. Words
   B. Music
   C. Graphics
   D. All of the above
3. A _____ is a computer that can solve complex scientific equations and may be used for worldwide weather forecasting.
   A. Supercomputer
   B. Mainframe
   C. Embedded computer
   D. Microcomputer
4. A _____ can generate a payroll for a large business. Several hundred users can access terminals at the same time.
   A. Supercomputer
   B. Mainframe
   C. Embedded computer
   D. Microcomputer

5. The type of input device, which collects data directly from the environment and sends it to the computer, is called a _____. It is used in clinical monitoring devices.
   A. Scanner
   B. Sensor
   C. Mouse
   D. Keyboard

6. Pointing devices include the _____.
   A. Mouse
   B. Trackball
   C. Light pen
   D. All of the above

7. An input device which reads printed text aloud is the _____.
   A. Keyboard
   B. Mouse
   C. Digitizing tablet
   D. Kurzweil scanner

8. The actual manipulation of data inside the computer is performed by the _____.
   A. Input devices
   B. Output devices
   C. Processing unit
   D. Secondary storage devices

9. Traditional phone lines are the slowest communications media. Comprised of two strands of copper, they are called _____.
   A. Twisted pair
   B. Coaxial cable
   C. Microwave communications
   D. Fiber optic cable

10. Which of the following are high-speed telecommunications lines?
    A. DSL
    B. ISDN
    C. T1
    D. All of the above

11. The fastest communications medium, _____, is made of thin strands of glass or plastic.
    A. Twisted pair
    B. Coaxial cable
    C. Microwave communications
    D. Fiber optic cable

12. Standards governing communications are called _____.
    A. Standards
    B. Protocols
    C. Conventions
    D. Rules

13. The _____ is a global network, which connects many smaller networks.
    A. Intranet
    B. Extranet
    C. Internet
    D. None of the above
14. The part of the Internet comprised of pages with hyperlinks to other pages is referred to as the _____.
    A. Public information utility
    B. Bulletin board system
    C. World Wide Web
    D. None of the above
15. The _____ directs the operation of the computer in accordance with the program's instructions.
    A. Arithmetic-logic unit
    B. Control unit
    C. Printer
    D. All of the above

True/False Questions

1. Embedded computers can be embedded in humans as well as appliances. _____
2. Information technology includes not only computers, but also networks and computer literacy. _____
3. Data and information are the same. _____
4. A computer manipulates data by following the step-by-step instructions of a program. _____
5. Hardware refers to the physical components of the computer. _____
6. Another word for hardware is programs. _____
7. Optical disks save data as pits and lands created by a laser. _____
8. The main circuit board of a computer is called the motherboard. _____
9. Application software controls the basic operations of the computer hardware including input and output. _____
10. The operating system must be booted for the computer to work. _____
11. If you are using a computer to create a budget, you would need a word processing program. _____
12. The binary number system uses two digits: 0 and 1. _____
13. Signals carried on traditional phone lines are analog waves. _____
14. A modem translates from digital to analog and analog to digital signals. _____
15. You are sure to get reliable medical information from the Web. _____

Critical Thinking

1. What input devices do you foresee being used in the health care field? Comment on how such devices as sensors and speech-recognition devices are especially relevant to your discipline.

2. What measures can be taken to help assure the quality of medical information one receives over the World Wide Web?

3. The World Wide Web has impinged on our lives in many ways. How has it affected your personal and professional (or academic) activities?

SOURCES

Anderson, Sandra. *Computer Literacy for Health Care Professionals.* Albany, NY: Delmar, 1992.

Austen, Ian. "A Scanner Skips the ID Card and Zeroes in on the Eyes." nyt.com (May 15, 2003; May 19, 2003).

Baase, Sara. *A Gift of Fire: Social, Legal, and Ethical Issues in Computing.* Upper Saddle River, NJ: Prentice-Hall, 1996.

Beekman, George. *Computer Confluence: Exploring Tomorrow's Technology,* 5th ed. Upper Saddle River, NJ: Prentice-Hall, 2002.

Bisdikian, Chatschik, and Brent Miller. "What Is Bluetooth?" http://www.informit.com/ (July 12, 2002; May 19, 2003).

Bond, Paul. "A-Listers Join 'Quest' for Kids with Asthma." http://www.hollywoodreporter.com (July 24, 2002; May 19, 2003).

Bureau of Labor Statistics Occupational Outlook Handbook 2002–2003. http://stats.bls.gov/ oco/ocos163.htm (2002–2003; May 19, 2003).

Divis, Dee Ann. "Bill Would Push Driver's License with Chip." *Insight on the News.* http://Insightmag.com (May 1, 2002; May 8, 2004).

Eisenberg, Anne. "When the Athlete's Heart Falters, a Monitor Dials for Help." nyt.com (January 9, 2003; January 9, 2003).

Feder, Barnaby. "Face-Recognition Technology Improves." nyt.com (March 14, 2003; March 14, 2003).

Fein, Esther B. "For Many Physicians, E-Mail Is the High-Tech House Call." *New York Times,* November 20, 1997, pp. A1, B8.

Harmon, Amy. "U.S., in Shift, Drops Its Effort to Manage Internet Addresses." *New York Times,* June 6, 1998, pp. A1, D2.

Markoff, John. "High-Speed Wireless Internet Is Planned." nyt.com (December 6, 2002; May 15, 2003).

Oakman, Robert L. *The Computer Triangle,* 2d ed. New York: Wiley, 1997.

Peterson, Melody. "Internet Ads Promising Cures or Protection." nyt.com (April 14, 2003; April 14, 2003).

Pogue, David. "Learning to Talk to Your PC." nyt.com (March 4, 2004; May 7, 2004).

Race, Tim. "What Do They Mean by Digital, Anyhow?" *New York Times,* March 19, 1998, p. G11.

Salamone, Salvatore. "VPN Eases Meetings of the Mind." *PC World,* June 15, 1998, pp. 1, 78.

Senn, James A. *Information Technology in Business: Principles, Practices, and Opportunities,* 2d ed. Upper Saddle River, NJ: Prentice-Hall, 1998.

Stewart, Angela. "Health Departments Will Link Up to Share Data." *Star-Ledger,* July 18, 1998.

RELATED WEB SITES

The following sample of Web sites can provide research information on medical matters. However, we cannot vouch for the accuracy of the information.

Healthfinder (http://www.healthfinder.gov) for a government listing of nonprofit and government organizations which can provide you with health-related information

PubMed (http://www.ncbi.nlm.nih.gov/PubMed) for access to reliable medical information databases

OncoLink (http://www.oncolink.upenn.edu) for information on cancer

HealthTouch Online (http://www.healthtouch.com) for information on medications

MedicineOnLine (http://www.meds.com) for infomation on pharmaceutical and medical device companies

U.S. National Library of Medicine (www.nlm.nih.gov/) . . . Health Information MEDLINE/PubMed, MEDLINEplus, NLM Gateway. Library Services Catalog, Databases, Historical Materials, MeSH, Publications . . . Description: The world's largest medical library

CHAPTER 2

Security and Privacy in an Electronic Age

OUTLINE

- **Learning Objectives**
- **Security and Privacy—An Overview**
- **Threats to Information Technology**
  - *Computer Technology and Crime*
  - *Security*
- **Privacy**
- **Databases**
  - *Government Databases*
  - *Private Databases*
  - *Databases and the Internet*
- **Privacy, Security, and Health Care**
  - *Health Insurance Portability and Accountability Act (HIPAA) of 1996*
  - *Privacy of Medical Records Under HIPAA and the USA Patriot Act*
  - *Telemedicine and Privacy*
  - *E-mail and Privacy*
  - *Privacy and Electronic Medical Records*
- **Chapter Summary**
- **Key Terms**
- **Review Questions**
  - *Multiple Choice*
  - *True/False Questions*
  - *Critical Thinking*
- **Sources**
- **Related Web Sites**

LEARNING OBJECTIVES

Upon completion of this chapter, you will be able to

- Define security and privacy.
- Discuss threats to information technology, including crimes, viruses, and the unauthorized use of data.
- Discuss security measures, including laws, voluntary codes of conduct, restriction of access to computer systems, and the protection of information on networks.
- Describe the impact of information technology on privacy, including the existence of large computerized databases of information kept by both government and private organizations, some of which are on networks linked to the Internet.
- Describe the relationship of privacy and security to health care, and appreciate the importance of the privacy of electronic medical records.
- Discuss the Health Insurance Portability and Accountability Act of 1996 (HIPAA) and the USA Patriot Act (2000), specifically their effects on privacy protections.

SECURITY AND PRIVACY—AN OVERVIEW

Information technology and the expansion of the Internet have changed the way we live. More and more institutions—schools, businesses, hospitals, government agencies—depend on computers. Computers enable them to collect, store, and process enormous amounts of information quickly and efficiently. At the same time, any harm to computer systems is more threatening to the normal conduct of business. Safeguarding computer systems becomes critical. Guaranteeing the accuracy and **security**, and protecting the **privacy** of electronic records, including medical records, is crucial. It is an ongoing challenge. In March 2003, the following appeared in *The Centre Daily Times* (Texas): "In Kentucky, state computers put up for sale as surplus . . . contained confidential files naming thousands of people with AIDs and sexually transmitted diseases. The oversight was discovered when the state auditor's office purchased eight of the computers. Thousands of state-owned computers may still be out there" (Mitchell, 2003).

Privacy has many aspects. Among them is the ability to control personal information and the right to keep it from misuse. Computer technology makes this much more difficult. Security measures attempt to protect computer systems, including information, from harm and abuse; the threats may stem from many sources, including natural disaster, human error, or crime including the spreading of **viruses**. Protection may take the form of anything from professional and business codes of conduct, to laws, to restricting access to the computer.

This chapter deals with threats to information technology, stressing dangers to the privacy of information in electronic databases as well as measures to protect the security of computer systems. The existence of massive government and private databases on the Internet poses dangers to personal privacy. The chapter also deals with computers and trends in health care delivery, including the growth of health maintenance organizations and medical insurance companies, the relationship of telemedicine to issues of privacy and security, the use of electronic medical records, and e-mail. The electronic sharing of medical records can help save lives by assuring continuity of care. However, the lack of security in computer systems in health care organizations and on networks in general endanger doctor-patient confidentiality and the privacy of medical information. Even under HIPAA, medical records are accessible not only to your physicians, but also to insurance companies, labs, pharmacies, and hospital clerical staffs. This chapter discusses attempts to make electronic medical records secure, including the first federal legislation protecting the privacy of medical records—the Health Insurance Portability and Accountability Act of 1996 (HIPAA).

THREATS TO INFORMATION TECHNOLOGY

Threats to information technology include hazards to hardware, software, networks, and to data, including information stored in electronic databases. **Data accuracy** and security are what is most relevant to the use of computerized medical records. However, computer hardware, software, and data can be damaged by anything from simple carelessness to power surges, crime, and computer viruses. Computer systems, like any other property, can be hurt or destroyed by such disasters as floods and fires.

Computer Technology and Crime

Computer technology has led to new forms of crime. Crimes involving computers can be crimes using computers and/or crimes against computer systems. Many times they are both—using computers to harm computer systems. Computer crime includes committing fraud and scams over the Internet, unauthorized copying of software protected by copyright (called **software piracy**), and **theft of services** such as cable TV. Software piracy costs the software industry billions of dollars a year. According to the Business Software Alliance, over 30 percent of software is pirated (Beekman, 2003, p. 314). **Theft of information**, including breaking into a medical database and gaining access to medical records, is also considered a crime.

One common computer crime is **fraud**—such as using a computer program to illegally transfer money from one bank account to another, or printing payroll checks payable to oneself. Fraudulent purchases over the Internet are common. Purchases over the Internet are increasing; 58 percent of them are purchases of hardware and software. A favorite target of Internet thieves is software. Since software is delivered instantly—electronically—it is sometimes received before credit card numbers are checked.

Viruses can also damage hardware, software, and data. A virus is a program that attaches itself to another program and replicates itself. A virus may do damage to your hardware or destroy your data, or it may simply flash an annoying message. Most states and the federal government make it a crime to intentionally spread a computer virus. Federal law makes it a felony to do $1,000 or more worth of damage to any computer involved in interstate commerce. This includes any personal computer connected to the Internet. The penalties for damaging computer systems have been severely increased by the USA Patriot and Homeland Security Acts. Spreading viruses is a kind of high-tech vandalism. Virus detection software can find and get rid of many but not all viruses.

One of the most valuable resources of any organization is data or information. An accurate list of a business's customers with their purchases and credit records, or of a doctor's patients with their confidential medical histories, is a vital asset that cannot be replaced. It is crucial that this information be correct and secure. However, this is not always the case. Data may be incorrect simply because of carelessness in data entry; that is, information in a database is erroneous due to faulty entry or an inaccurate source. However, data may be correct and still vulnerable to misuse. Some information, including medical records, is highly personal and subject to abuse. Protecting the privacy of records kept on electronic databases and on networks is extremely difficult, if not impossible.

Identity theft involves someone using your private information to assume your identity. It is the fastest growing crime in the United States. Although identity theft predates computers, the existence of computer networks, the centralization of information in databases, and the posting of public information on the Internet make information much easier to steal. An identity thief needs only a few pieces of information (such as your Social Security number or your mother's maiden name) to steal your identity. Under this false identity—your identity—the thief can take out credit cards, loans, buy houses, and even commit crimes. Identity theft is extremely difficult to prosecute. It is also not easy for the victim to correct all the negative information that the thief has created. False negative information may keep appearing in response to every routine computer check. Currently some cities are putting all public records, including property and court records, on the Internet, making identity theft even easier to commit. Think of the information (including your signature) on the ticket you were issued last month.

Security

Security measures attempt to protect computer systems and the privacy of computerized data. They can include anything from laws and **codes of conduct** to restricting access to computers, to **encryption**—scrambling of data so that it does not make sense. There are federal laws which attempt to protect computer systems and aspects of privacy.

There are also codes of conduct within some businesses and organizations, which attempt to safeguard information. Protecting privacy on the Internet is a much more difficult problem. In December 1997, in order to forestall government regulation, several computer companies and look-up services reached agreement on a code of conduct to limit public access to personal data on the Internet. The code would allow people to have their names removed from databases, but it includes no way of informing people what is online about them or giving them a way to correct it. A person would have to contact all fourteen companies and ask to have his or her name removed from each database. The agreement also would ask marketers to "voluntarily limit the collection of personal data." Encryption would be used to protect private information. Social Security numbers, mother's maiden name, birth date, credit and financial records, and medical records would no longer be available to the general public; private investigators and law enforcement agencies would have access to this information.

Federal Legislation on Computers and Privacy

1970—Fair Credit Reporting Act regulates credit agencies. It allows you to see your credit reports to check the accuracy of information and challenge inaccuracies.

1974—Privacy Act prohibits disclosure of government records to anyone except the individual concerned, except for law enforcement purposes. It also prohibits the use of information except for the purpose for which it was gathered. It deals with the use and disclosure of Social Security numbers.

1978—Right to Financial Privacy Act establishes procedures for the federal government to follow when looking at bank records.

1984—Computer Fraud and Abuse Act prohibits unauthorized access to federal computers.

1986—Electronic Communications Privacy Act prohibits government agencies from intercepting electronic communications without a search warrant. It also prohibits individuals from intercepting e-mail. However, there are numerous exceptions and the courts have interpreted this to allow employers to access employees' e-mail. This law does not apply to communications within an organization.

1988—Video Privacy Protection Act prohibits video rental stores from revealing what tapes you rent.

1988—Computer Matching and Privacy Protection Act limits the use of computer matching.

1994—Computer Abuse Amendments Act makes it a crime to "gain unauthorized access to a computer system [used in interstate commerce] with the intent to obtain anything of value, to defraud the system, or to cause more than $1000 worth of damage." This applies to *any* computer linked to the Internet. It specifically prohibits the transmission of viruses.

1996—National Information Infrastructure Protection Act establishes penalties for interstate theft of information and for threats against networks and computer system trespassing.

1996—Health Information Portability and Accountability Act puts a national floor under privacy protections for medical information.

1997—Driver Privacy Protection Act limits disclosure of personal information in Motor Vehicles records.

2000—Children's Online Privacy Protection Act requires Web sites targeting children aged 13 or under to get parental consent to gather information on the children.

2001—The USA Patriot Act gives law enforcement agencies greater power to monitor electronic and other communications, with fewer checks.

2002—The Homeland Security Act expands and centralizes the data gathering allowed under the Patriot Act.

(continued)

Many other acts, introduced in the 107th Congress, are presently in committee:

2001—Online Privacy Protection Act to require the Federal Trade Commission to issue regulations protecting the privacy of personal information collected on the Internet.

2001—Social Security Online Privacy Protection Act to regulate the use of Social Security and other personally identifiable information by interactive computer services.

2001—Electronic Privacy Protection Act would prohibit the sale of any information collection device without proper labeling or notice.

2001—Consumer Internet Privacy Enhancement Act would protect the privacy of consumers using the Internet.

2001—Fair Credit Reporting Act Amendments of 2001 would further protect consumers from the negative consequences of inaccurate consumer credit reports.

2001—Personal Information Privacy Act would protect the privacy of individuals with respect to personal information.

2001—Confidential Information Protection Act would protect the privacy of information acquired for statistical purposes.

2001—Video Voyeurism Act would prohibit video voyeurism in the maritime and territorial jurisdiction of the United States.

Adapted from June Parsons and Dan Oja, et al., *Computers, Technology, and Society* (Cambridge, MA: ITP, 1997), PRV-14-15; Larry Long and Nancy Long, *Computers,* 5th ed. (Upper Saddle River, NJ: Prentice Hall, 1998), Issues-19; Gary Shelley and Thomas Cashman, *Discovering Computers: A Link to the Future* (Cambridge, MA: Thomson Course Technology, 1997), 13.21; "Driver Privacy Protection Act," http://www/state.ma.us/rmv/privacy.index.htm; Global POV (March 28, 2003); Arter and Hadden—IP Newsletter: Privacy Law Update (February 2001; March 28, 2003); "EFF Analysis of the Provisions of the USA Patriot Act That Relate to Online Activities" (October 31, 2001), eff.org (October 31, 2001; April 11, 2003); David Holtzman, "Homeland Security and You," CNET news.com (January 21, 2003; April 23, 2003).

Many organizations restrict access to their computers. This can be done by requiring authorized users to have **PINs (personal identification numbers)** or use **passwords**. Locking computer rooms and requiring employees to carry ID cards and keys are also used to restrict access. **Biometric methods**, including **fingerprints, hand prints, retina** or **iris scans, lip prints, facial thermography**, and **body odor sensors**, also help make sure only authorized people have access to computer systems. Biometric technology can use facial structure to identify individuals. **Biometric keyboards** can identify a typist by fingerprints. None of these methods is foolproof. Even biometric methods, which for a time were seen as more reliable, are far from perfect. PINs and passwords can be forgotten or shared, and ID cards and keys can be lost or stolen. Biometric methods also pose a threat to privacy, since anyone who can gain access to the database of physical characteristics, gains access to other, possibly private information about you. Some biometric measures are inherently different than other security measures. In more traditional methods, such as fingerprinting, you are aware that your identity is being checked. However, iris and retina scans, facial thermographs, **facial structure scans**, and body odor sensors allow your identity to be checked without your knowledge, cooperation, or consent. This can be seen as an invasion of privacy.

Since more than one-half of computer frauds are committed internally, by authorized employees (Beekman, 2003, p. 312), restricting access to authorized employees may do little good. An overwhelming majority of information security managers in private, government, and university settings believe that "disgruntled employees were the most likely cause of data security incidents." Developing company policy and codes of conduct and making sure that all employees are aware of them might be a first step toward security.

Protecting information that is kept on a network is much more difficult because no one knows who can access a network. Even top-secret defense systems have been broken into. One way of protecting data is through encryption. Only authorized persons can see the decrypted data. Electronic blocks (called **firewalls**) can be used to limit access to networks. None of these measures guarantees security; therefore, a protection plan that includes backing up data is always necessary. This guarantees that you have an accurate copy of the data you need, but does nothing to protect data from misuse.

PRIVACY

Computer technology has transformed the way we assemble, store, and protect data, including highly confidential material. It has also changed the way we work at jobs. Almost every white-collar worker has a microcomputer on his or her desk. The personal computer has replaced the typewriter. E-mail is replacing the memo and phone call. This makes both our words and our work more subject to scrutiny and less private. People think of e-mail as private; it is not. According to Barry Lawrence of the Society of Human Resource Management, "e-mail [is] like a postcard. Anyone can read it along the way." Employees are fired for using e-mail for private communications or for sending messages critical of their bosses. The **Electronic Communications Privacy Act of 1986** has been interpreted to allow employers access to employees' e-mail. Not only are your words subject to scrutiny but also your work is scrutinized. When you are working on your office PC, every keystroke may be monitored and counted by your employer.

As an employee, you have a very restricted right to privacy. In 1977, the Federal Privacy Protection Commission, under pressure from business groups, did not ask Congress to make it a crime for employers to gather information "unrelated to job performance" about employees. As a consumer, when you make a purchase with a credit card, your name, address, and credit card number, along with your purchases, are recorded. The information becomes part of your credit history, and a profile of your buying habits can be put together and sold to direct marketers. Records that used to be kept in physically separate places—your credit history in one store's credit file, or your health records in your doctor's office, or a city's records of births, marriages, and vehicle ownership in a county courthouse—are now organized in databases, stored on computers, linked to networks, available to anyone with a computer and a modem.

Smart cards are currently being used in many states as driver's licenses. These cards can contain information about the driver and links to government and private databases. In May 2002, the Driver's License Modernization Act was introduced in Congress. It would standardize state licenses. Every license would include an ID chip. Because the chip would be programmable, it would replace ATM and credit cards and other identification cards. Supporters of the cards maintain that the smart card would be harder to counterfeit than the licenses used today and therefore protect individuals against identity theft. They also maintain that by making licenses an identity card, it would enhance national security. They point to the low cost and convenience of being able to carry just one card, instead of a credit card, an ATM card, and a driver's license. Privacy advocates warn of the danger of a unique identifier, which could be used by businesses to build a specific and detailed picture of a consumer. They further warn that the electronic codes protecting the cards cannot really be secure.

Computer technology and the Internet allow for the inexpensive and easy gathering and distribution of personal information—from the most mundane to the most intimate details of our lives—which may be collected without our consent or knowledge. Laws have been proposed to create some minimal privacy rights on the Internet; for example, some sites now have to get parental consent before collecting information from children. The computer may gather information about you without your knowledge as you browse the Net. **Cookies** are small files that a Web site may put on your hard drive when you visit. Cookies can be programmed to track your movements, collecting information that helps advertisers target you. This information may be sold and shared; the fact is that you do not control your information once it is in cyberspace.

DATABASES

An electronic **database** is an organized collection of data that is easy to access, manipulate, search, and sort. Gathering facts is not new. A decennial census is mandated by the U.S. Constitution, so that representation in Congress can be determined. Records of birth, marriage, death, divorce, property ownership, taxes, driving, and bankruptcy are all on file. The local library even keeps records of the books you check out until they are returned. These records were always kept. However, they used to be kept in the local courthouse or motor vehicles department—every file physically and logically separate from every other file. To access the records, you had to travel to where the file was kept. Today, with the use of computerized databases on networked computers, this is not the case. Through the use of Social

Security numbers as identifiers, the information in one database can be linked to information in other databases and a complete and detailed portrait of any individual can be painted.

Government Databases

Large databases of information are kept by the federal and local governments, as well as by private businesses. Agencies of the federal government maintain more than 2,000 databases. The FBI's National Crime Information Center includes 24 million records. The Internal Revenue Service (IRS) keeps a database on the source and amount of income we earn and the taxes we pay. The Social Security Administration has records used to determine your eligibility for benefits. The Department of Defense has a database, which includes your draft status. The National Directory of New Hires is a new database that the federal government was required to start on October 1, 1997, by the 1996 welfare law. Every time a person is hired, his or her name must be reported along with address, Social Security number, and wages. Wage reports are required every three months. The data collected by the Census Bureau is now computerized, although by law it cannot be used against a respondent.

Agencies of the government may use computer matching to link data in several databases. For example, the IRS uses computer matching to match tax records with vehicle registration and other records kept by state governments and with private records of large transactions kept by banks. The IRS looks for expensive purchases such as cars and boats and for large cash transactions. The National Directory of New Hires is matched against the Department of Health and Human Services' list of everyone owing or owed child support, and the lists are checked against each other. Some federal agencies (including the IRS, Social Security Administration, and Secret Service) use computer profiling—a technique that puts together a portrait of a person "likely" to commit a crime. Computer profiling is also being used by the government's Computer-Assisted Passenger Screening Program, which "uses several dozen criteria, all but a few secret, to screen for the air travelers most likely to be drug lords or terrorists." Although data gathered by the government is subject to some regulation, data gathered by private companies is not. Government and private companies do cooperate in the gathering of data. Currently, certain jurisdictions are putting all their records online. This means your signature is available on a traffic ticket, and the details of your divorce can be read like a novel.

Since September 11, 2001, Congress, concerned with security, passed two bills that effect privacy: the USA Patriot Act (2001) and the Homeland Security Act (2002). The **USA Patriot Act** gives law enforcement agencies greater power to monitor electronic and other communications, with fewer checks. It allows increased sharing of information between the states, the FBI, and the CIA. The law expands the authority of the government to allow roving wiretaps, which intercept communications, wherever the person is. Both e-mail and voice mail may be seized under a search warrant (Plesser, 2002). The government may track Web surfing and request information from Internet service providers about their subscribers. The law is establishing a DNA database that will include anyone convicted of a violent crime. Some of these provisions are currently scheduled to sunset or expire in 2005.* However, the **Homeland Security Act** expands and centralizes the data gathering allowed under the Patriot Act. A new federal department of Homeland Security is established to analyze data collected by other agencies. The law includes expanded provision for the government to monitor electronic communications and authority for the government to mine databases of personal information at the same time that it limits congressional oversight. Any government body at any level can now request information from your ISP without a warrant or probable cause, as long as there is a "good faith" belief that national security is involved. Your local library is required to turn over any records to the FBI, if asked. The act limits an individual's access to information under the Freedom of Information Act. If a business states that its activities are related to security, that information will be kept secret (Weinstein, 2002). The law gives government committees more freedom to meet in secret. It limits liability for companies producing antiterrorism products, including vaccinations, at the same time that the government would gain wider power to declare national health emergencies, quarantines, and order forced vaccinations.

The most far-reaching proposal of all is called the **Total Information Awareness Program**. However, Congress has put this program on hold. TIAP would allow the mining of databases and e-mail for information on Americans, including financial, credit, health, purchasing, travel, telephone, and other data. Software would be used to look for "patterns" suggesting terrorist activity. The results of government and business surveillance would be linked.

Private Databases

Private organizations keep computerized databases of employees and potential customers. Hospitals keep records of patients. You may not be aware that data is being gathered or that the data gathered may be entered in a database. The information in the databases may be available to the general public over the Internet. Unaware of the existence of the information, you have no opportunity to check its accuracy. When you buy something using a credit card at the supermarket, fill out a warranty card, subscribe to a magazine, fill out a survey questionnaire, or rent a movie, data is collected about your purchasing habits. When you make a phone call, a record is kept of the phone number, time, and length of the call. All this information is collected for commercial purposes; businesses can buy your profile and analyze it, looking for likely customers. However, you do not control what happens to information about you or who will become aware of the brand of soap you use in the shower.

The **Medical Information Bureau** is of particular interest. It is comprised of 650 insurance companies. Its database contains the health histories of 15 million people. The information in this huge database is used by medical insurers to help determine insurance rates and whether to grant or deny medical coverage. The medical histories in this database are not protected by doctor-patient privilege, but may gain some

*For a complete list of these provisions, see "EFF Analysis of the Provisions of the USA Patriot Act That Relate to Online Activities" (October 31, 2001), eff.org (October 31, 2001; April 11, 2003).

protection under the Health Insurance Portability and Accountability Act of 1996 (HIPAA).

Credit bureaus receive information from businesses and banks. From this they compile a credit history and credit report. Your credit report is used as a basis for granting or denying you a credit card, mortgage, or student loan. It may also be requested by a potential employer and may be used to deny you a job. Although the use and content of credit reports is regulated by the **Fair Credit Reporting Act of 1970**, it is extremely difficult to remove inaccurate negative information.

Some private companies (data warehouses) exist for the sole purpose of collecting and selling personal information. They sell information to credit bureaus and to employers for background checks. Since September 11, 2001, the demand for background checks on prospective (or even current) employees has increased. One company experienced a 33 percent increase in the demand for background checks. The linking of information is making these background checks more thorough. Electronic databases are now being linked into larger and more comprehensive super databases. For example, in November 2001, one company linked together criminal records from all U.S. jurisdictions (a database of 20 million convictions). Before that, each jurisdiction had to be searched separately. "To test the system, ChoicePoint decided to run a batch of names from previous screenings. One of the names . . . had been submitted by a client who had requested a criminal search only locally . . . No convictions showed up. But when the name was entered into the new nationwide database of criminal convictions this fall . . . records were located in Tennessee. 'One was for murder, one for grand theft.'" (Guernsey, 2001).

Databases and the Internet

When files were first computerized, they were kept in separate computer systems; security could be as easy as locking the door to the computer room and requiring each authorized user to have valid identification. Today computerized files are kept on networks; many are linked to the Internet. The information includes such highly personal data as Social Security numbers, dates of birth, mothers' maiden names, and unlisted phone numbers. Companies such as Lexis-Nexis and Equifax sell credit and financial information and other records to banks, insurance companies, and direct marketers. You have no way of knowing what information is available about you, what organization's database it is in, or of seeing it or checking its accuracy. The impact of this is serious. Anyone with access to your Social Security number can gain access to information about you and even assume your identity.

PRIVACY, SECURITY, AND HEALTH CARE

The privacy of medical records is something people are very concerned about. Several trends combine to threaten the security and privacy of health care information. First, health care information has traditionally been protected by state law. Now, however, this information routinely crosses state lines, which means it needs federal protection.

It is very difficult to protect information on computer networks, especially the Internet. The privacy protections of the Health Information Portability and Accountability Act of 1996 began going into effect on April 14, 2003. HIPAA provides the first federal protection for the privacy of medical records.

Health Insurance Portability and Accountability Act (HIPAA) of 1996

Given the facts of current medical practice—the use of the electronic medical record stored on networks, telemedicine, and information that routinely crosses state lines—federal protection has become a necessity.

In 1996, Congress passed the **Health Insurance Portability and Accountability Act (HIPAA).** Guidelines to protect electronic medical records were developed by the Department of Health and Human Services. By encouraging the use of the electronic medical record and facilitating the sharing of medical records among health care providers, it can assure continuity of care and thus save lives. If you are in an accident far from home, the availability of your medical history can prevent medical catastrophes such as allergic reactions to medications. However, the more easily your records are available, the less secure they are. Medical information can be used against you. According to a report by the U.S. Congress, it is crucial to safeguard the privacy of health information since "[i]naccuracies in the information or its improper disclosure, can deny an individual access to . . . basic necessities of life, and can threaten an individual's personal and financial well-being" (Protecting Privacy of Medical Information, January 21, 2003, page 5).

HIPAA "encourag[es] electronic transactions, but it also requires new safeguards to protect the security and confidentiality" of health information (HHS Fact Sheet, March 9, 2001). The new safeguards do not override stronger state protections. For the first time, all patients have the right to see their medical records and the right to *request* changes. Patients will have some knowledge of the use of their medical records and must be notified in writing of their providers' privacy policy. HIPAA gives patients more control over their medical information. Under the rule, medical records must be supplied within 30 days of the patient's request, and the patients are allowed to review and copy their own records as they wish. Prior to HIPAA, many states did not give patients the legal right to see their records. Additionally, the patient can request amendments be made to their records if their appeal is justifiable.

HIPAA regulations began going into effect on April 14, 2001. Health plans, clearinghouses, and providers who use electronic billing and funds transfer had until April 14, 2003, to comply. Other entities have until April 2006 to comply. The new regulations cover "[a]ll medical records and other individually identifiable health information used or disclosed by a covered entity in any form, whether electronically, on paper, or orally." Higher standards apply to psychotherapy notes, which are not considered part of a medical record under this law, and "are never intended to be shared with anyone else." The law applies to both public and private providers and institutions. Providers must give patients a written explanation of how their health information may be used; patients may see, copy, and *request* changes in their medical records. Providers need to make a good faith effort to get a patient's consent before using his or her information. Health information may no longer be used by employers or banks to make decisions regarding employment or loans. Except for the sharing of information for the purpose of treatment, payment, or business operations, "disclosures . . . will be limited to the minimum necessary" (HHS Fact Sheet, March 9, 2001). In practice this may mean that any health care business can see personal health information with little regard for treatment.

Health care providers and institutions may design their own procedures to meet the new standards; however, they must be written and must include the following information: who has access to patient information, how this information will be used, and the conditions under which it may be shared. Health care providers are responsible for seeing that those with whom they do business also protect patient privacy. Employees must be trained to respect patient privacy and follow privacy procedures, and one person must be chosen to ensure that the privacy procedures are followed. Under specific conditions, health information may be shared without the patient's consent (e.g., for public health needs, research, and some law enforcement activities, and when the interests of national defense and security are involved). Under HIPAA, violations of the law can be punished by both civil and criminal penalties (HHS Fact Sheet, March 9, 2001).

Some of the original privacy protections have been weakened, for example, the requirement of a patient's written consent for disclosure of health information ("Final Modifications to the HIPAA Privacy Regulations," 2002). Because of this, some privacy advocates stress the weaknesses of the privacy protection. According to James Pyles, a lawyer from Washington, D.C., "Almost any health care business can now have access to personal health information if it can show that the information is needed for treatment, payment or business operations" (Mitchell, 2003). However, with all its weaknesses, HIPAA will provide the first national minimum privacy protections for health information (HHS Fact Sheet, March 9, 2001).

Privacy of Medical Records under HIPAA and the USA Patriot Act

Under both HIPAA and the Patriot Act, there are many circumstances that allow police access to your medical records without a warrant. HIPAA allows the release of private medical information in some situations, including the assertion that you are a suspect or witness to a crime or a missing person. Your information may also be released if national security or intelligence is involved or for the protection of VIPs, including the president and foreign dignitaries. The government may also access your medical records under the USA Patriot Act "for an investigation to protect against international terrorism or clandestine intelligence activities" (Section 215). HIPAA requires that you be informed in a general way how your records may be used without consent. However, you do not have to be notified of any specific sharing of your information, and further the USA Patriot Act does not allow you to be told. Because

HIPAA and the USA Patriot Act are so new, the constitutionality of the provisions that allow warrantless access has not been tested.

Telemedicine and Privacy

Telemedicine refers to any kind of health care administered over telecommunications lines. This would include the use of e-mail by physicians to communicate with patients and colleagues, distance exams and consultations, teleradiology, and telepsychiatry, among other specialties. Health care information, comprised of medical records, live videos, psychiatric consultations, and radiologic images has traditionally been protected by state regulations. But now this information routinely crosses state lines. Therefore, HIPAA protection is of special importance. HIPAA requires that e-mail be secured either by using encryption or controlling access. HIPAA specifically discusses privacy issues of telemedicine, including the presence of nonmedical personnel (e.g., camera people and other technicians) and the fact that the more stringent privacy protection (federal or state) has precedence (Telehealth Update: Final HIPAA Privacy Rules, February 20, 2001).

E-mail and Privacy

For some doctors and their patients, e-mail is becoming a common form of communication. It is used as a practical, easy, inexpensive way of confirming or changing appointments, asking and answering questions, and maintaining communication over long distances. Some physicians also see it as a way to rebuild the traditional personal doctor-patient relationship that existed prior to managed care. Some doctors see e-mail as an intimate form of communication. However, e-mail has not been private. It is not like a phone conversation; a permanent record of e-mail communications exists. Although e-mail is private in transit, it is not protected while stored. As mentioned, courts have ruled that employers have the legal right to read employees' e-mail, and today many doctors are employees of health maintenance organizations. E-mail may be read on any of the computer systems it passes through on its way between doctor and patient. Because of the threats to the privacy of medical information, many doctors are now refusing to use e-mail. The requirements of HIPAA that e-mail be encrypted may help with these issues.

Privacy and Electronic Medical Records

Your medical records include information about your total physical and mental makeup. They may discuss your relationships with family members, sexual behavior, and drug or alcohol-related problems. One particularly sensitive piece of information is one's HIV status. On a personal level, knowing that anyone has access to intimate details of your life may be humiliating.

Computerizing medical records and making them easily available over networks is, of course, essential to good medical care and can save lives. However, access to networked medical records is not limited to medical personnel. The issues of privacy and the easy availability of records kept on networked databases have special impact on health care and medical ethics. Most people assume the confidentiality of the doctor-patient relationship. This confidentiality is challenged by several trends. The movement to computerize medical records and possibly put them on the Internet, the expanding use of telemedicine, the use of e-mail by health care workers, the increased use of health maintenance organizations, and reliance on third parties to pay for medical care all raise serious questions of patient confidentiality and medical ethics. Under HIPAA, however, health care providers and their business associates have put some privacy protections in place.

A National Research Council report issued in March 1997 found that although electronic medical records are becoming more and more common, they were not secure and little was being done to protect them. The report stated that certain precautions can be taken to limit access to medical records. However, six years later medical records were still not secure. In March 2003, less than one month before HIPAA required privacy protection of medical records, Texas reported that the computer network shared by 16 state agencies and 225 private and public organizations lacked protection for medical records. Some proposed protections include requiring the use of passwords by authorized users, using electronic blocks (called firewalls) to limit the access to networks, and keeping track of who actually sees a record through audit trails. The most obvious precaution is to train personnel not to leave patient information displayed on a computer screen.

Many people now receive health care through health maintenance organizations. Under managed care, people are seen by several health care providers and records are shared. For example, a patient seen by a general practitioner can be referred to a gastroenterologist for an MRI and blood work. The patient's records are seen by primary care physicians, hospital and lab personnel, radiologists, pharmacists, consultants, and office staffs. Patients' records are also available to state health organizations and researchers. This electronic paper trail is then monitored by the health insurance provider, and may be seen by an employer seeking to cut medical insurance costs. "Most patients would be surprised at the number of organizations that receive information about their health record," according to Dr. Paul D. Clayton of Columbia Presbyterian Medical Center in New York and chair of the National Research Council Panel. Dr. Clayton is only referring to authorized users. Incidents have occurred in which unauthorized users (**hackers**) have gained access to hospital computer systems and changed patient information. The possibility of theft of patient information also exists.

There are presently proposals to put medical records on the Internet. The first attempt at storing electronic medical records on the Internet took place at the University of California at San Diego School of Medicine. Ideally, both patients and health care providers would be able to see their records wherever they can access the Internet. The biggest problem is security. They are trying to institute privacy protection, while allowing authorized health care providers access. The security systems used to protect medical records on the Internet will be similar to security systems used by defense and military installations. Those designing this security recognize that "nothing in cyberspace is impregnable."

CHAPTER SUMMARY

Chapter 2 introduces the reader to the issue of security for computer systems and the importance of the privacy of the information on those systems—specifically medical records. Although guaranteeing the privacy of medical records was always important, keeping these records on databases on networks raises new problems.

- Threats to information technology may stem from many sources, including crime, viruses, human error, and natural disaster.
- Security measures that attempt to protect computer systems including information, may include laws, codes of conduct, encryption, and restricting access. Restricting access may be done by assigning PINs or passwords, requiring ID cards and keys, or through biometric methods. Firewalls (electronic blocks to access) may be used to protect information on networks.
- Computer technology changes the nature of the way we work, and makes work more subject to scrutiny.
- The Internet makes gathering personal information easy and inexpensive.
- The existence of networked databases of personal information, especially if they are connected to the Internet, endangers privacy by making that information accessible to anyone.
- HIPAA provides the first national standards for the privacy and security of health information. Under HIPAA and the USA Patriot Act, there are many instances when government agencies can access your medical records.

KEY TERMS

biometric keyboards
biometric methods
body odor sensors
codes of conduct
cookies
data accuracy
database
Electronic Communications Privacy Act of 1986
encryption
facial structure scans
facial thermography
Fair Credit Reporting Act of 1970

fingerprints
firewalls
fraud
hackers
hand prints
Health Insurance Portability and Accountability Act (HIPAA)
Homeland Security Act
identity theft
iris scans
lip prints
Medical Information Bureau

passwords
personal identification numbers (PINs)
privacy
retina scans
security
software piracy
theft of information
theft of services
Total Information Awareness Program
USA Patriot Act
viruses

REVIEW QUESTIONS

Multiple Choice

1. Threats to information technology include threats to _____.
   A. Hardware
   B. Software
   C. Data
   D. All of the above

2. The unauthorized copying of software protected by copyright is called _____.
   A. Theft of services
   B. Software piracy
   C. A and B
   D. None of the above

3. Breaking into a medical database and gaining access to medical records is an example of a crime called _____.
   A. Theft of services
   B. Theft of information
   C. Software piracy
   D. Network piracy

4. Which of the following is a way of attempting to protect computer systems and data from unauthorized use?
   A. Encryption
   B. Codes of conduct
   C. Restricting access through the use of PINs
   D. All of the above

5. Biometric security methods include _____.
   A. Use of passwords
   B. Locking the computer room
   C. Iris scans, lip prints, and body odor sensors
   D. Carrying ID cards

6. Using a computer to create a description of someone who, you believe, is "likely" to commit a crime is called _____.
   A. Computer matching
   B. Computer profiling
   C. Computer graphics
   D. None of the above

7. Privacy means _____.
   A. The ability to control personal information and keep it from misuse
   B. The attempt to protect computer hardware from criminals
   C. The attempt to protect computer hardware from natural disaster
   D. None of the above

8. Threats to information technology may stem from _____.
   A. Crime
   B. Human error
   C. Natural disaster
   D. All of the above
9. A program that attaches itself to another program, replicates itself, and may do damage to your computer is called a _____.
   A. Network
   B. Database
   C. Virus
   D. None of the above
10. Computer crimes include _____.
    A. Software piracy
    B. Theft of services such as cable TV
    C. Theft of information
    D. All of the above
11. The first federal protection for the privacy of medical information is provided by the _____.
    A. Homeland Security Act
    B. Health Insurance Portability and Accountability Act
    C. USA Patriot Act
    D. All of the above
12. The _____ gives law enforcement agencies greater power to monitor electronic and other communications, with fewer checks.
    A. Health Insurance Portability and Accountability Act
    B. Privacy Act
    C. USA Patriot Act
    D. All of the above
13. _____ are small files that a Web site may put on your hard drive when you visit. They can be programmed to track your movements, collecting information that helps advertisers target you.
    A. Cookies
    B. Tracers
    C. A and B
    D. None of the above
14. _____ limits disclosure of personal information in motor vehicles records.
    A. Driver Privacy Protection Act
    B. Motor Vehicle Act
    C. Federal Privacy Act
    D. None of the Above
15. The _____ has a database that contains health histories of millions of people.
    A. Immigration and Naturalization Service (INS)
    B. Medical Information Bureau (MIB)
    C. National Crime Information Center (NCIC)
    D. None of the above

True/False Questions

1. Most computer frauds are committed by employees of the organization being defrauded. _____
2. E-mail is a private communication. _____
3. According to the Electronic Privacy Information Center, most Web sites have privacy policies. _____
4. Computer matching links the information in one database to the information in other databases. _____
5. The Medical Information Bureau contains medical records of millions of people, and it guards the privacy of these records. _____
6. Traditionally, health care information has been protected by state law. _____
7. Computerizing medical records and making them available over networks helps facilitate sharing of medical records among health care providers and, therefore, can help assure continuity of care. _____
8. Medical records on the Internet are guaranteed to be secure. _____
9. Hackers have never gained access to hospital computer systems. _____
10. It is a crime for employers to gather information about their employees. _____
11. Under HIPAA, medical records get some federal privacy protection. _____
12. Under some circumstances, government agencies have access to your medical information without a warrant. _____
13. There is a federal proposal to use smart cards as drivers' licenses. _____
14. Under HIPAA, health information may still be used by employers or banks to make decisions regarding employment or loans. _____
15. Under HIPAA, you have the right to examine your medical records. _____

Critical Thinking

1. Assume that the information you provide when you register as a college student is kept in a networked database. This includes personal details such as your name, Social Security number, birth date, address, financial and marital status, and prior educational records. How would you safeguard the privacy of this information?
2. Numerous medical organizations are keeping records online. Some are linking their hospital networks to the Internet. How would you propose protecting the confidentiality of the doctor-patient relationship in this situation?
3. Proposals have been made to use smart cards as driver's licenses. Using one identifying number, the license could gain access to other information contained in private and government databases. The license could also function to replace your credit card and ATM card. List the advantages and disadvantages of using smart cards as driver's licenses.
4. Computer profiling is being used to identify people "likely" to commit a crime. Although these people are not automatically arrested, they may be stopped and questioned for no reason other than their profile "fits." In a democracy, people are supposed to be arrested only after a crime is committed, and even then they are presumed innocent. Does computer profiling violate these tenets of democracy?

5. Where would you draw the line on how much private information (e.g., name, Social Security number, mother's maiden name, unlisted phone number and address, financial and medical information) should be available on the Internet? What are the pros and cons of government regulation?
6. Discuss why privacy and security are especially important issues in the new millennium.
7. How do HIPAA and the USA Patriot Act affect the privacy of medical information? Does the possible loss of privacy guarantee greater national security?

SOURCES

"Answers to Frequently Asked Questions about Government Access to Personal Medical Information (under the USA Patriot Act and the HIPAA regulations)." American Civil Liberties Union, www.aclu.org (May 30, 2003; June 18, 2003).

Arter and Hadden. IP Newsletter: Privacy Law Update. arterhadden.com (February 2001; March 28, 2003).

Austen, Ian. "A Scanner Skips the ID Card and Zooms in on the Eyes." nyt.com (May 15, 2003; May 16, 2003).

Baase, Sara. *A Gift of Fire: Social, Legal, and Ethical Issues in Computing.* Upper Saddle River, NJ: Prentice-Hall, 1996.

Beekman, George. *Computer Confluence: Exploring Tomorrow's Technology,* 5th ed. Upper Saddle River, NJ: Prentice-Hall, 2003.

Bernstein, Nina. "Personal Files via Computer Offer Money and Pose Threat." *New York Times,* June 12, 1997, pp. A1, B14.

Center for Telemedicine Law. Legislative Action. ctl.org (2002; May 15, 2003).

Chaddock, Gail Russell. "Security Act to Pervade Daily Lives." *Christian Science Monitor,* csmonitor/2002/1121/p01s03-usju.html (November 21, 2002; March 31, 2003).

Clymer, Adam. "Conferees in Congress Bar Using a Pentagon Project on Americans." nyt.com (February 12, 2003; February 12, 2003).

"Congress Debates National Drivers License with ID Tracking Chip" May 1, 2002, DOJgov.net, *Newswire,* http://www.dojgov.net/national_license-01.htm (May 1, 2002; May 6, 2003).

Cronin, Anne. "Census Bureau Tells Something about Everything." *New York Times,* December 1, 1997, p. D 10.

Donovan, Larry. "Privacy Law Update." http://library.lp.findlaw.com (2001; March 27, 2003).

"EFF Analysis of the Provisions of the USA Patriot Act That Relate to Online Activities (October 31, 2001)." eff.org (October 31, 2001; April 11, 2003).

Electronic Privacy Information Center. Latest News. epic.org (May 6, 2003; May 6, 2003).

Electronic Privacy Information Center. "Medical Record Privacy." http://www.epic.org/privacy/medical (March 28, 2002; May 14, 2003).

Feder, Barnaby. "Face-Recognition Technology Improves." nyt.com (March 14, 2003; March 14, 2003).

Fein, Esther B. "For Many Physicians, E-mail Is the High-Tech House Call." *New York Times,* November 20, 1997, pp. A1 and B8.

"Final Modifications to the HIPAA Privacy Regulations."
http://www.hallrender.com/pdf000551HA.pdf (2002; March 27, 2003).

Fitzgerald, Thomas J. "A Trail of Cookies? Cover Your Tracks." nyt.com (March 27, 2003;
March 27, 2003).

Glass, Andrew. "Computer Industry Adopts Internet Privacy Code." *PR NEWSWIRE*.
http://nytsyn.com, pp. 1–2 (1997; December 28, 1997).

Global POV. http://www.globalpov.com/ (n.d.; March 28, 2003).

Guernsey, Lisa. "What Did You Do before the War?" nyt.com (November 22, 2001; March 28,
2003).

Hafner, Katie. "Why Doctors Don't E-mail." nyt.com (June 6, 2002; August 30, 2002).

Harrison, Ann. "Behind the US Patriot Act." AlterNet.org (November 5, 2001; April 11,
2003).

"HIPAA Detail: Email Security," Washington, D.C.
http://www.ioma.org/pdf/hipaa/hipaaemailsecurity.pdf (Summer 2001; May 15, 2003).

Holtzman, David. "Homeland Security and You." CNETNews.com (January 21, 2003;
April 23, 2003).

HHS Fact Sheet. hhtp://ssps.hhs.gov/admissimp/final/profact2.htm (March 9, 2001;
January 10, 2002).

Leary, Warren E. "Panel Cites Lack of Security on Medical Records." *New York Times,*
March 6, 1997, pp. A1, B11.

Lee, Jennifer. "Dirty Laundry, Online for All to See." nyt.com (September 5, 2002;
September 5, 2002).

———. "Finding Pay Dirt in Scannable Driver's Licenses." nyt.com (March 21, 2002;
March 24, 2002).

———. "Identity Theft Complaints Double in '02." nyt.com (January 22, 2003; January 23,
2003).

Lewis, Peter H. "Forget Big Brother." *New York Times,* March 19, 1998, pp. G1, G6.

Lichtblau, Eric. "Republicans Want Terror Law Made Permanent." nyt.com (April 9, 2003;
April 9, 2003).

Markoff, John. "Guidelines Don't End Debate on Internet Privacy." *New York Times,*
December 18, 1997.

McCullagh, Declan. "Bush Signs Homeland Security Bill." CNETNews.com (November 25,
2002; April 23, 2003).

Mitchell, Mitch. "Medical Privacy Law Stirs Controversy." *Star Telegram.* dfw.com (March 3,
2003; October 15, 2003).

Murphy, Dean E. "Librarians Use Shredder to Show Opposition to New F.B.I. Powers."
nyt.com (April 7, 2003; April 7, 2003).

Newman, Andy. "Face-Recognition Systems Offer New Tools, but Mixed Results." nyt.com
(May 3, 2001; August 30, 2002).

Parsons, June, Dan Oja, et al. *Computers, Technology, and Society.* Cambridge, MA: ITP, 1997.

Pear, Robert. "Bush Acts to Drop Core Privacy Rule on Medical Data." nytimes.com
(March 22, 2002; March 22, 2002).

———. "Health System Warily Prepares for Privacy Rules." nyt.com (April 6, 2003; April 6,
2003).

———. "Vast Worker Database to Track Deadbeat Parents." *New York Times,* September 22,
1997.

Plesser, Ronald L., et al. "*1 USA Patriot Act for Internet and Communications
Companies." http://cyber.law.harvard.edu (March 2002; May 8, 2004).

Plesser, Ronald L., James J. Halpert, and Emilio W. Ciridanes. "Summary and Analysis of Key Sections of the USA Patriot Act of 2001." piperruddnick.com (2001; May 18, 2004).

"Protecting Privacy of Medical Information." p. 5. http://www.mit.gov.in/telemedicine. (January 21, 2003; May 8, 2004).

Reuters. "Senate Rebuffs Domestic Spy Plan." *Wired News.* www.reuters.com (January 23, 2003; March 30, 2003).

Safire, William. "You Are a Suspect." nyt.com (November 14, 2002; March 31, 2003).

Schwaneberg, Robert. "Questions Leave 'Smart Card' in Limbo for Now." *Star-Ledger,* June 30, 1998, pp. 11, 14.

———. "Smart Cards Take a Step in Legislature." *Star-Ledger,* June 23, 1998, pp. 11, 15.

Schwartz, John. "Threats and Responses: Planned Databank on Citizens Spurs Opposition in Congress." nyt.com (January 16, 2003; March 26, 2003).

Seelye, Katharine Q. "A Plan for Database Privacy, but Public Has to Ask for It." *New York Times,* December 18, 1997, pp. A1, A24.

Shelley, Gary, and Thomas Cashman. *Discovering Computers: A Link to the Future,* Cambridge, MA: ITP, 1997.

Slater, Eric. "Biometric Revolution Aids Security, but Has Dark Side." *Star Ledger,* June 1, 1998, p. 41.

"Surfer Beware: Personal Privacy and the Internet." Report of the Electronic Privacy Information Center, Washington, D.C. http://www.epic.org/Reports/surfer-beware.html (June 1997; October 9, 2003).

"Telehealth Update: Final HIPAA Privacy Rules." http://telehealth.hrsa.gov/pubs/hipaa.htm (February 20, 2001; May 15, 2003).

"Telemedicine Licensing and Legislation." http://www.unc.edu (n.d.; May 14, 2003).

Wayner, Peter. "Code Breaker Cracks Smart Cards' Digital Safe." *New York Times,* June 22, 1998, pp. D1–D2.

Weinstein, Lauren. "Taking Liberties with Our Freedom." *Wired News.* wired.com (December 2, 2002; March 31, 2003).

RELATED WEB SITE

Electronic Privacy Information Center (http://www.epic.org) is a research organization concerned with privacy issues. It keeps a Privacy Archive with "an extensive collection of documents, reports, news items, policy analysis and laws relating to privacy issues."

An Introduction to Medical Informatics and the Administrative Applications of Computers

OUTLINE

- **Learning Objectives**
- **Medical Informatics**
- **Administrative Applications of Computer Technology in the Medical Office**
- **Medical Office Administrative Software—An Overview**
  - *The Patient Information Form*
  - *The Electronic Medical Record*
  - *Coding and Grouping*
- **Accounting, Using MediSoft**
- **Insurance**
  - *Claims*
- **Accounting Reports**
- **Other Systems**
- **Chapter Summary**
- **Key Terms**
- **Review Questions**
  - *Definitions*
  - *Multiple Choice*
  - *True/False Questions*
  - *Critical Thinking*
- **Sources**

LEARNING OBJECTIVES

Upon completion of this chapter, you will be able to

- Define medical informatics.
- Define clinical, special purpose, and administrative applications of computer technology in health care and its delivery.

- Define telemedicine.
- Discuss the computerization of tasks in the medical office with specific reference to MediSoft.
  - Describe the electronic medical record.
  - Define bucket billing.
  - Discuss coding and grouping systems, insurance, and the various accounting reports used in the medical office.
- Discuss coding and grouping systems used in other health care environments.

MEDICAL INFORMATICS

Medical informatics is a rapidly expanding discipline. It has a 30-year history in which it has sought to improve the way medical information is managed and organized. Medical informatics is located at the "intersection of information technology and . . . medicine and health care" (Gennari, 2002). Medical informatics has many definitions. The common emphasis in all definitions of medical informatics is on the use of technology to organize information in health care. That information includes patient records, diagnostics, expert systems, and therapy. The stress is not on the actual application of computers in health care, but the theoretical basis. Medical informatics is an interdisciplinary science "underlying the acquisition, maintenance, retrieval, and application of biomedical knowledge and information to improve patient care, medical information, and health science research." The tool used to perform these tasks is the computer (Gennari, 2002). The goal of medical informatics is the improvement of health care. Some of the problems medical informatics focuses on include improving the clarity of diagnostic images, improving image-guided and minimally invasive surgery, developing simulations that allow health care workers to improve treatments without practicing on human subjects, developing low-cost diagnostic tests, treating physical handicaps, providing consumers with information, coordinating international medical reporting, developing and improving information systems used in health care settings, and developing decision-support systems. The application of computer technology continues to contribute to the achievement of these goals.

Traditionally the application of computer technology in health care is divided into three categories. The **clinical applications** of computers include anything that has to do with direct patient care, such as diagnosis, monitoring, and treatment. **Special purpose applications** include the use of computers in education and some aspects of pharmacy. **Administrative applications** include office management, scheduling, and accounting tasks. MediSoft and other programs like it are specifically designed for medical office management. **Telemedicine**—the delivery of health care over telecommunications lines—includes clinical, special purpose, and administrative applications. Chapters 4 through 11 deal in detail with clinical and special purpose applications of computer technology. This chapter explores how computers have transformed administrative tasks in the medical office.

ADMINISTRATIVE APPLICATIONS OF COMPUTER TECHNOLOGY IN THE MEDICAL OFFICE

Beginning with the computerization of hospital administrative tasks in the 1960s, the role of digital technology in medical care and its delivery has expanded at an ever-increasing pace. Today computers play a part in every aspect of health care.

As you recall, administrative applications include office management tasks, scheduling, and accounting functions. These are tasks that need to be performed in any office. However, some of these activities are slightly different in a health care environment, so programs are needed that take into account the special needs of a health care environment. There are many programs that automate and computerize functions in health care environments. Some are for doctors' offices; some are for dentists. Others are for hospitals, emergency rooms, pharmacies, or chiropractors. Some are off-the-shelf commercial software; others are written specifically for a particular office or hospital. All these programs attempt to automate practice management from the initial scheduling of an appointment, to diagnosis, to the electronic processing of insurance claims, and bucket billing (billing each insurance company and then the patient in a timely manner). These programs make it possible to keep track of a patient's billing and health status electronically. The needs of each type of health care setting of course differ. For example, in a hospital setting, programs need to deal with admission, discharge, and transfer. Because there are so many different programs that accomplish similar tasks, we have chosen to describe one commercial program in detail.

MediSoft is one of the many programs specifically designed to computerize basic administrative functions in a health care environment—the coding and grouping systems, insurance information, and payment information. It allows the user to organize information by patient, by case, and by provider. It enables the user to schedule patient appointments with a computer; take electronic progress notes; create lists of codes for diagnosis, treatment, and insurance; submit claims to primary, secondary, and tertiary insurers; and receive payment electronically. MediSoft is appropriate to the **bucket billing** that medical offices must use to accommodate two or three insurers, who must be billed in a timely fashion before the patient is billed. Moreover, because MediSoft is a **relational database** (an organized collection of related data), information input in one part of the program can be linked to information in another part of the program. Billing information and financial status are easily available in MediSoft. Tables can be searched for any information, and this information can be presented in finished form in one of the many report designs provided, including various kinds of billing reports. If no report design meets the user's need, a customized report can easily be designed and generated by the user. MediSoft software can be used by medical administrators and office workers, doctors and other health care workers, and students. It can ease the tasks of administering a practice using a computer. The amount of data and information a modern practice has to collect and organize is overwhelming. MediSoft allows the user to computerize tasks performed every day in any medical environment. All the disparate tasks and pieces

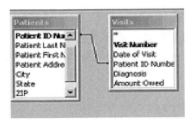

FIGURE 3.1 In a relational database, such as one created using Microsoft Access®, tables can be related using a common field. Two tables (one for patient information and one for visit information) are linked using Patient ID Number, the common field. Many tables in one database file can be linked.

of data and information need to be well organized, accessible, and easily linked. Because MediSoft is a relational database, the user can quickly and easily organize, access, and link information from one part of the program to information in any other part of the program.

A **database** is an organized collection of information. A **database management system (DBMS)** allows the user to enter, organize, and store huge amounts of data and information. The information can then be updated, sorted, resorted, and retrieved. In order to use database management software efficiently, the user should be familiar with certain concepts and definitions. A database **file** holds all related information on an entity, for example, a medical practice. Within each file, there can be several **tables**. Each table holds related information. For example, one table might hold information on a practice's doctors; another holds information on its patients; another on its insurance carriers. A table is made up of related **records**; each record holds all the information on one item in a table, that is, one patient. Each patient has a record in the practice's patient table. All the information on one patient makes up that patient's record. Each record is made up of related **fields**. One field holds one piece of information, such as a patient's last name, or Social Security number, or chart number. One field—the **key** field—uniquely identifies each record in a table. The information in that field cannot be duplicated. Social Security number is a common key field because no two people have the same SSN. Chart number uniquely identifies each patient's chart. MediSoft is also a relational database in which related tables are linked by sharing a common field (see Figure 3.1).

MEDICAL OFFICE ADMINISTRATIVE SOFTWARE—AN OVERVIEW

Medical office administration software, such as MediSoft, allows the user to create one database file for each **practice** (group of medical practitioners in business together). Within each database, information is organized in tables. The tables are linked by sharing a common field.

The Patient Information Form

At or before a patient's first visit, he or she fills out a patient information form, which includes such personal data as name, address, home and work phones, date of birth, Social Security number, and student status. The patient is also asked to fill in information about his or her spouse or partner.

Medical information is required: allergies, medical history, and current medications. The patient is also asked for the reason for the visit, such as accident or illness, and the name of a referring physician.

In addition, the patient is asked to provide insurance information for him- or herself and a spouse or partner. This information includes the name of the primary, secondary, and tertiary insurance carriers, name and birth date of the policyholder, the copayment, and policy and group numbers.

The Electronic Medical Record

The information that was gathered and entered onto a patient information form is then entered into a computer. This forms the patient's medical record. Encouraged by HIPAA, the **electronic medical record (EMR)** is replacing the paper record. Documentation of medical conditions and treatments is going online. The EMR may be stored in a hospital's private network, but it also may be kept on the Internet. There are many benefits to the EMR. Because your record is available anywhere there is a computer on the network, the EMR helps guarantee continuity of care. Each of your health care providers knows your full medical history and can therefore provide better care. If you are in an accident in New Jersey, for example, but live in California, your record is a mouse-click away. The EMR is legible and complete. Despite its benefits, the EMR raises serious privacy and financial issues. Any network can be broken into, and your medical information can be stolen and misused; a great deal of medical information is private. No one wants their psychiatric diagnosis, HIV status, or children's head lice broadcast to the neighborhood. HIPAA (the Health Insurance Portability and Accountability Act of 1996) is providing the first federal protection for medical records. (See Chapter 2 for a full discussion of HIPAA and the privacy of medical information.) Introducing the EMR can cost $10,000 per year per doctor. In an effort to cut costs, the federal **Centers for Medicare and Medicaid Services (CMS)**, formerly the **Health Care Financing Administration (HCFA)**, has recommended the development of an open source EMR—free to physicians and fully customizable. One is being developed by the American Academy of Family Physicians. Critics assert that this will not solve all the problems of the EMR and that most health care professionals are not proficient enough with computers to customize the software.

Proposals have been made to put electronic medical records on smart cards—cards that include a computer chip and can hold a great deal of information. However, in the United States the use of smart cards has not progressed far beyond the pilot project stage (Hagland, 2000). The use of the card has been hampered by security and privacy concerns. The card has certain benefits to the patient and the practitioner. Patients would have all their medical information available for emergencies.

Coding and Grouping

Each of these categories of information (personal, medical, insurance) is entered onto a form and becomes part of a record in a table in a database. Some of it is translated into codes before it is entered. Codes provide standardization, which allows the easy sharing of information. Because codes of diagnoses and procedures are precise and universally used, one physician can recognize another's diagnoses and procedures immediately.

A standard grouping system is **DRG (diagnosis related group)**. Today, hospital reimbursement by private and government insurers is determined by diagnosis. Each patient is given a DRG classification, and a formula based on this classification determines reimbursement. If hospital care and cost exceed the prospective cost determination, the hospital absorbs the financial loss.

Services including tests, lab work, exams, and treatments are coded using **CPTs** (*Current Procedural Terminology*, 4th ed.). **ICD-9-CM** provides three-, four-, or five-digit codes for thousands of diseases. The ICD is the *International Classification of Diseases Clinical Modification*, 9th ed. These coding systems make electronic claims forms easier to file because each condition or disease, each service, procedure, and diagnostic test can be identified by a widely agreed-on code number. These codes are standardized, but no practice uses all of them. When a new practice is set up, only codes that relate to its specialty are entered in one of the tables of codes; these tables can always be amended. The CPT is used on the **superbill** or **encounter form** (list of diagnoses and procedures common to the practice) to identify all procedures performed by that specialty (see Figure 3.3 on page 50).

ACCOUNTING, USING MEDISOFT

MediSoft is essentially an accounting program. Therefore, several definitions are required. **Charges, payments**, and **adjustments** are called **transactions**. A charge is simply the amount a patient is billed for the provider's service. A payment is made by a patient or an insurance carrier to the practice. An adjustment is a positive or negative change to a patient account. Transactions are organized around cases. A **case** is the condition for which the patient visits the doctor. This information is entered by the medical office staff and stored in the practice's database tables. There can be several visits associated with one case. The case can be closed when the condition is resolved. And there can be several cases (one for each diagnosis) for one patient.

INSURANCE

Today, many people are covered by medical insurance. Those people who are not covered either pay out-of-pocket or seek care in the local emergency room. A **guarantor** is the person responsible for payment; it may be the patient or a third party. There are a variety of options for those with insurance. Some carriers have a **schedule of benefits**—a list of those services that the carrier will cover. This is called an **indemnity plan**. Indemnity plans are becoming less and less common, because they are **fee-for-service plans**, and therefore very expensive. The patient is never restricted to a network of providers and needs no referrals for specialists. After fulfilling a **deductible** (a certain amount the patient is required to pay each year before the insurance begins paying,) every visit to a doctor is paid for by the insurance company. The doctor, not the insurance company, determines necessary care and treatment so there is no financial reason for a health care worker to deny necessary care. **Managed care** also has a schedule of benefits for out-of-network providers. Managed care plans and **preferred provider organizations (PPOs)** may require that the provider get **authorization** before a procedure is performed. This is simply permission by the insurance carrier for the provider to perform a medical procedure.

A patient with PPO insurance can seek care within an approved network of health care providers who have agreed with the insurance company to lower their charges and accept **assignment** (the amount the insurance company pays). The patient may pay a **copayment**, the part of the charge for which the patient is responsible. The patient may choose, however, to go out-of-network and pay the provider's customary charges. The insurance company may then reimburse the patient a small amount.

There are several government insurance plans. They are administered by the federal Centers for Medicare and Medicaid Services (CMS), formerly the Health Care Financing Administration (HCFA). Seventy-four million Americans receive their health care through government insurers—some through fee-for-service plans, some through managed care (U.S. Department of Health & Human Services, 2003). According to HHS, **Medicaid** is "jointly funded, federal-state health insurance for certain low-income and needy people. It covers approximately 36 million individuals including children, the aged, blind, and/or disabled, and people who are eligible to receive federally assisted income maintenance payments." Medicaid resembles managed care in that the patient is restricted to a network of providers, must get a preauthorization for procedures, and needs referrals to any specialist. **Medicare** serves people 65 and over and disabled people with chronic renal disorders. Medicare allows patients to choose their physicians; referrals are not needed. Some Medicare patients choose to belong to HMOs. Many people supplement Medicare with private fee-for-service plans in which they are not restricted to a network of providers; they do not need referrals to specialists. The patient is required to pay a cost-sharing amount; the provider bills the insurance for the remainder. **CHAMPVA** and **TRICARE** are federal health benefits programs that supplement medical care in the military. **Workers' compensation** is a government program that covers job-related illness or injury.

With managed care, it is the insurance carrier that determines what treatment is necessary and pays for it. There are several forms of managed care. In managed care, patients pay a fixed yearly fee, and the insurance company pays the participating provider.

A patient who uses a **health maintenance organization (HMO)** pays a fixed yearly fee, and must choose among an approved network of health care providers and hospitals. The patient needs a referral from his or her primary care provider to see any specialist. If a patient goes out-of-network without the HMO's approval, the patient must pay out-of-pocket. However, this may change in light of a Supreme Court decision of April 2, 2003. Under the ruling, states may require HMOs to open their networks, allowing patients more choice.

In a **capitated plan**, a physician is paid a fixed fee (the capitation), and the physician is paid regardless of the amount of treatment he or she provides. Some patients may seek no treatment; some may visit several times.

Claims

To receive payment for services from an uninsured patient, the practice simply bills the patient. To receive payment for services rendered to an insured patient, the practice must submit a **claim** to the insurance carrier. A claim is a request to an insurance company for payment for services. If an insurance carrier requires a treatment plan, the current version of MediSoft enables you to create one. There are many claim forms, but the most widely accepted form is the **HCFA-1500** (see Figure 3.2). (Because of the change in name of HCFA to CMS, the name of the form is currently being changed to **CMS-1500** [www.cms.hhs.gov/forms].) It is accepted by government insurers and most private plans. An **EMC (electronic media claim)** is an electronically processed and transmitted claim.

To create a claim to submit to an insurance company, the practice needs to gather certain information: the patient's condition, the physician's diagnosis, and the procedures performed in the office or hospital. The patient record can provide them with personal data, medical history, and insurance information. The provider table can supply information about the physician. Claims are submitted on paper or electronically. Practices that submit electronic claims use a **clearinghouse**—a business that collects insurance claims from providers and sends them to the correct insurance carrier. An insurance company can reject the claim, or send a check for partial or full payment. The response to a paper claim includes an **explanation of benefits (EOB)** which explains why certain services were covered and others not; an **electronic remittance advice (ERA)** accompanies the response to an EMC. The practice records the claim and applies it to the charge. It then bills the secondary insurer; the EOB from the first insurer is sent to the secondary insurer with the bill. The secondary insurer responds with a check and EOB or ERA. After the response is received from the secondary insurer, the tertiary insurance company is billed. It is only after the response is received from all of a patient's carriers

PLEASE
DO NOT
STAPLE
IN THIS
AREA

CARRIER

PICA

HEALTH INSURANCE CLAIM FORM

PICA

1. MEDICARE	MEDICAID	CHAMPUS	CHAMPVA	GROUP HEALTH PLAN	FECA BLK LUNG	OTHER	1a. INSURED'S I.D. NUMBER	(FOR PROGRAM IN ITEM 1)
(Medicare #)	(Medicaid #)	(Sponsor's SSN)	(VA File #)	(SSN or ID)	(SSN)	(ID)		

2. PATIENT'S NAME (Last Name, First Name, Middle Initial)

3. PATIENT'S BIRTH DATE MM DD YY   SEX M F

4. INSURED'S NAME (Last Name, First Name, Middle Initial)

5. PATIENT'S ADDRESS (No., Street)

6. PATIENT RELATIONSHIP TO INSURED
Self Spouse Child Other

7. INSURED'S ADDRESS (No., Street)

CITY | STATE

8. PATIENT STATUS
Single Married Other

CITY | STATE

ZIP CODE | TELEPHONE (Include Area Code) ( )

Employed Full-Time Student Part-Time Student

ZIP CODE | TELEPHONE (INCLUDE AREA CODE) ( )

9. OTHER INSURED'S NAME (Last Name, First Name, Middle Initial)

10. IS PATIENT'S CONDITION RELATED TO:

11. INSURED'S POLICY GROUP OR FECA NUMBER

a. OTHER INSURED'S POLICY OR GROUP NUMBER

a. EMPLOYMENT? (CURRENT OR PREVIOUS)
YES NO

a. INSURED'S DATE OF BIRTH MM DD YY   SEX M F

b. OTHER INSURED'S DATE OF BIRTH MM DD YY   SEX M F

b. AUTO ACCIDENT?   PLACE (State)
YES NO

b. EMPLOYER'S NAME OR SCHOOL NAME

c. EMPLOYER'S NAME OR SCHOOL NAME

c. OTHER ACCIDENT?
YES NO

c. INSURANCE PLAN NAME OR PROGRAM NAME

d. INSURANCE PLAN NAME OR PROGRAM NAME

10d. RESERVED FOR LOCAL USE

d. IS THERE ANOTHER HEALTH BENEFIT PLAN?
YES NO   If yes, return to and complete item 9 a-d.

READ BACK OF FORM BEFORE COMPLETING & SIGNING THIS FORM.
12. PATIENT'S OR AUTHORIZED PERSON'S SIGNATURE I authorize the release of any medical or other information necessary to process this claim. I also request payment of government benefits either to myself or to the party who accepts assignment below.

SIGNED _____ DATE _____

13. INSURED'S OR AUTHORIZED PERSON'S SIGNATURE I authorize payment of medical benefits to the undersigned physician or supplier for services described below.

SIGNED _____

PATIENT AND INSURED INFORMATION

14. DATE OF CURRENT: ILLNESS (First symptom) OR INJURY (Accident) OR PREGNANCY(LMP) MM DD YY

15. IF PATIENT HAS HAD SAME OR SIMILAR ILLNESS. GIVE FIRST DATE MM DD YY

16. DATES PATIENT UNABLE TO WORK IN CURRENT OCCUPATION MM DD YY FROM TO MM DD YY

17. NAME OF REFERRING PHYSICIAN OR OTHER SOURCE

17a. I.D. NUMBER OF REFERRING PHYSICIAN

18. HOSPITALIZATION DATES RELATED TO CURRENT SERVICES MM DD YY FROM TO MM DD YY

19. RESERVED FOR LOCAL USE

20. OUTSIDE LAB? $ CHARGES
YES NO

21. DIAGNOSIS OR NATURE OF ILLNESS OR INJURY. (RELATE ITEMS 1,2,3 OR 4 TO ITEM 24E BY LINE)
1. _____   3. _____
2. _____   4. _____

22. MEDICAID RESUBMISSION CODE   ORIGINAL REF. NO.

23. PRIOR AUTHORIZATION NUMBER

24. A DATE(S) OF SERVICE From MM DD YY To MM DD YY	B Place of Service	C Type of Service	D PROCEDURES, SERVICES, OR SUPPLIES (Explain Unusual Circumstances) CPT/HCPCS	MODIFIER	E DIAGNOSIS CODE	F $ CHARGES	G DAYS OR UNITS	H EPSDT Family Plan	I EMG	J COB	K RESERVED FOR LOCAL USE
1											
2											
3											
4											
5											
6											

25. FEDERAL TAX I.D. NUMBER   SSN EIN

26. PATIENT'S ACCOUNT NO.

27. ACCEPT ASSIGNMENT? (For govt. claims, see back) YES NO

28. TOTAL CHARGE $

29. AMOUNT PAID $

30. BALANCE DUE $

31. SIGNATURE OF PHYSICIAN OR SUPPLIER INCLUDING DEGREES OR CREDENTIALS (I certify that the statements on the reverse apply to this bill and are made a part thereof.)

32. NAME AND ADDRESS OF FACILITY WHERE SERVICES WERE RENDERED (If other than home or office)

33. PHYSICIAN'S, SUPPLIER'S BILLING NAME, ADDRESS, ZIP CODE & PHONE #

PHYSICIAN OR SUPPPLIER INFORMATION

FIGURE 3.2   HCFA-1500 form.
Used by permission of MediSoft.

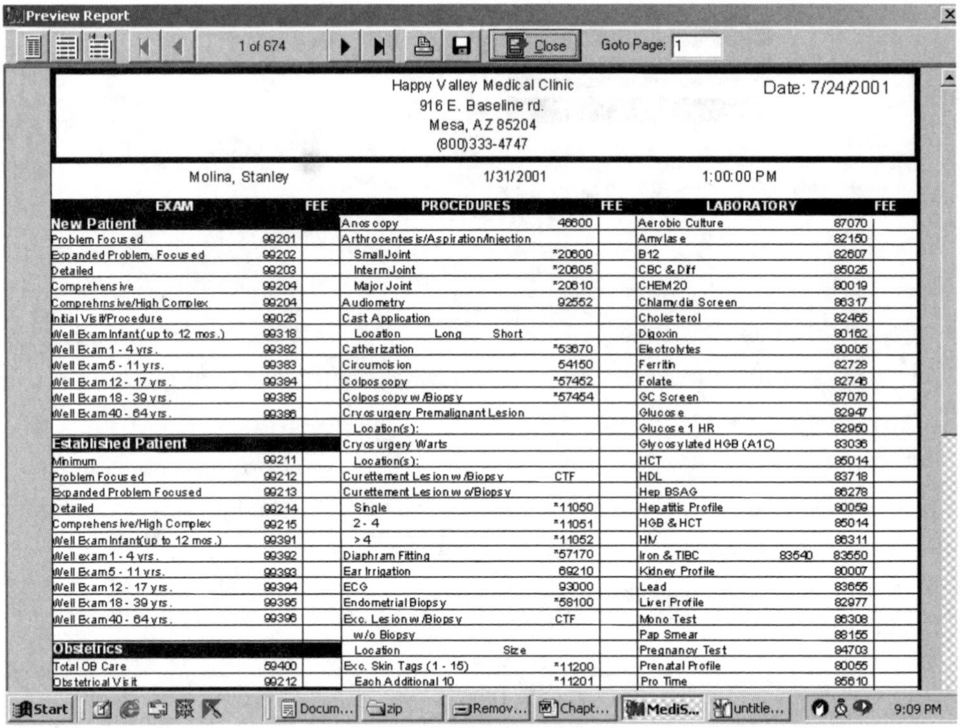

Happy Valley Medical Clinic
916 E. Baseline rd.
Mesa, AZ 85204
(800)333-4747

Date: 7/24/2001

Molina, Stanley 1/31/2001 1:00:00 PM

EXAM		FEE	PROCEDURES		FEE	LABORATORY		FEE
New Patient			Anoscopy	46600		Aerobic Culture	87070	
Problem Focused	99201		Arthrocentesis/Aspiration/Injection			Amylase	82150	
Expanded Problem, Focused	99202		Small Joint	*20600		B12	82607	
Detailed	99203		Interm Joint	*20605		CBC & Diff	85025	
Comprehensive	99204		Major Joint	*20610		CHEM20	80019	
Comprehrnsive/High Complex	99204		Audiometry	92552		Chlamydia Screen	86317	
Initial Visit/Procedure	99025		Cast Application			Cholesterol	82465	
Well Exam Infant(up to 12 mos.)	99318		Location Long Short			Digoxin	80162	
Well Exam 1 - 4 yrs.	99382		Catherization	*53670		Electrolytes	80005	
Well Exam 5 - 11 yrs.	99383		Circumcision	54150		Ferritin	82728	
Well Exam 12 - 17 yrs.	99384		Colposcopy	*57452		Folate	82746	
Well Exam 18 - 39 yrs.	99385		Colposcopy w/Biopsy	*57454		GC Screen	87070	
Well Exam 40 - 64 yrs.	99386		Cryosurgery Premalignant Lesion			Glucose	82947	
			Location(s):			Glucose 1 HR	82950	
Established Patient			Cryosurgery Warts			Glycosylated HGB (A1C)	83036	
Minimum	99211		Location(s):			HCT	85014	
Problem Focused	99212		Curettement Lesion w/Biopsy	CTF		HDL	83718	
Expanded Problem Focused	99213		Curettement Lesion w/o Biopsy			Hep BSAG	86278	
Detailed	99214		Single	*11050		Hepatitis Profile	80059	
Comprehensive/High Complex	99215		2 - 4	*11051		HGB & HCT	85014	
Well Exam Infant(up to 12 mos.)	99391		>4	*11052		HIV	86311	
Well exam 1 - 4 yrs.	99392		Diaphram Fitting	*57170		Iron & TIBC	83540 83550	
Well Exam 5 - 11 yrs.	99393		Ear Irrigation	69210		Kidney Profile	80007	
Well Exam 12 - 17 yrs.	99394		ECG	93000		Lead	83655	
Well Exam 18 - 39 yrs.	99395		Endometrial Biopsy	*58100		Liver Profile	82977	
Well Exam 40 - 64 yrs.	99396		Exc. Lesion w/Biopsy	CTF		Mono Test	86308	
			w/o Biopsy			Pap Smear	88155	
Obstetrics			Location Size			Pregnancy Test	84703	
Total OB Care	59400		Exc. Skin Tags (1 - 15)	*11200		Prenatal Profile	80055	
Obstetrical Visit	99212		Each Additional 10	*11201		Pro Time	85610	

FIGURE 3.3 Page 1 of a superbill created using MediSoft.
Used by permission of MediSoft.

that the patient is billed. This is called bucket billing or **balance billing**. MediSoft is structured to handle bucket billing, which is unique to the health care environment.

From the time a patient is charged for a procedure to the time when all payments have been received and credited to the patient's account, there is a sequence of accounting events that occur. **Accounts receivable (A/R)** include any invoices or any payment from the patient or insurance carriers to the medical practice. The diagnoses and procedures relevant to a patient's visit are recorded on a superbill (also called an encounter form) (see Figure 3.3). A superbill is a list of diagnoses and procedures common to the practice. Superbills for each patient on a day's schedule are printed that morning or the night before. Information taken from the superbill is utilized in several MediSoft accounting reports.

ACCOUNTING REPORTS

MediSoft provides the user with various kinds of reports that are generated on a daily, monthly, or yearly basis. Daily reports include a **patient day sheet**, a **procedure day sheet**, and a **payment day sheet**. A patient day sheet lists the day's patients, chart numbers, and transactions. It is used for daily reconciliation. A procedure day sheet is a grouped report organized by procedure. Patients who underwent a particular procedure, such as a blood sugar lab test, are listed under that procedure. This report is used to see what procedures a health care worker is performing. It also can be used to find the most profitable procedures. A payment day sheet is a grouped report organized by providers. Each patient is listed under his or her provider. It shows the amounts received from each patient to each provider (Burke and Weill, 2004, pp.126–129).

A **practice analysis report** is generated on a monthly basis, and is a summary total of all procedures, charges, and transactions (Burke and Weill, 2004, pp. 131–132).

A **patient aging report** is used to show a patient's outstanding payments. Current and past due balances are listed on this report based on the number of days late. For example, an account can be past due 30–60 days, 60–90 days, and over 90 (Burke and Weill, 2004, pp. 132–134).

The administrative and accounting tasks of a health care environment can be computerized using MediSoft. It allows the user to enter all necessary information into tables, link the information, and present it in one of the many reports it provides. Computerizing the accounting transactions allows the office to avoid being buried in paper, and keeps all accounts in an accurate, up-to-date, and well-organized structure.

OTHER SYSTEMS

Other types of health care facilities, such as skilled nursing facilities and hospitals, use different programs for organization and accounting. Hospital administrative programs have to take account of admission, transfer, and discharge. Some hospitals create their own programs. Many coding systems were developed in response to the Balanced Budget Act of 1997. This act mandated prospective payment systems for home health agencies, hospital outpatient care, and rehabilitation hospitals. For skilled nursing facilities, **resource utilization groups (RUGs)** were established. The system bases payment on average prices, with adjustments (Deparle, 1999). Using resident assessment instruments called **minimum data sets**, each patient is assigned to one of seven categories of RUG. Reimbursement for hospital outpatient services is based on **ambulatory patient classification (APC)**. The payment scales (Medicare Benefits Schedule) are developed based on relative value studies, which establish relative value scales. The scale can be developed using several measures such as current doctors' fees or doctors' assessment of the procedure's worth.

Other grouping and coding systems are also in use. **Healthcare Common Procedure Coding Systems (HCPCS)** were developed to standardize claims processing for government and private insurance. The system is divided into three subsystems: The first is a coding system identifying services and procedures. The second identifies products, supplies, and some services and equipment used outside the doctors' office. The third is comprised of codes developed by states.

HHRG (Home Health Resource Group) helps determine prospective payment for home health care for Medicare patients. HHRG is based on estimates determined by data collection using **OASIS (Outcome and Assessment Information Set)**. Based on HHRG each patient is assigned to one of 80 categories based on the severity of the patient's condition, functional status of the patient, and the use of services (OASIS Brochure http://www.cthomecare.org/OASIS%20Brochure%20-%20CT.pdf).

CHAPTER SUMMARY

Computers are used throughout our society, including the field of health care and its delivery.

Medical informatics has to do with the use of computers in the management and organization of medical information. Administrative applications include the use of computers in the medical office. Clinical applications use computers in such direct patient care as diagnosis, monitoring, and treatment. Special purpose applications include drug design and educational uses.

Telemedicine is the delivery of health care over telecommunications lines, and includes administrative, clinical, and special purpose applications.

Programs such as MediSoft allow the user to computerize medical office management functions.

- The electronic medical record is replacing the paper record.
- Bucket billing (or balance billing) is specific to health care office environments, where each insurer must be billed and payment received before the patient is billed.
- In today's medical office coding systems are used to identify conditions, tests, and procedures.
- Various types of insurance need to be understood.
- Different kinds of accounting reports are used in the medical office.
- Different types of care facilities use different programs and grouping and coding systems.

KEY TERMS

accounts receivable (A/R)
adjustments
administrative applications
ambulatory patient classification (APC)
assignment
authorization
balance billing
bucket billing
capitated plan
case
Centers for Medicare and Medicaid Operations (CMS)
CHAMPVA
charges
claim
clearinghouse
clinical application
CMS-1500
copayment
CPT (*Current Procedural Terminology*)
database
database management system (DBMS)
deductible
DRG (diagnosis related group)

electronic medical record (EMR)
electronic remittance advice (ERA)
EMC (electronic media claim)
encounter form
explanation of benefits (EOB)
fee-for-service plans
fields
file
guarantor
HCFA-1500
Health Care Financing Administration (HCFA)
health maintenance organization (HMO)
Healthcare Common Procedure Coding Systems (HCPCS)
HHRG (Home Health Resource Group)
ICD-9-CM (*International Classification of Diseases Clinical Modification*)
indemnity plan
key
managed care

Medicaid
medical informatics
Medicare
MediSoft
minimum data sets
OASIS (Outcome and Assessment Information Set)
patient aging report
patient day sheet
payment day sheet
payments
practice
practice analysis report
preferred provider organization (PPO)
procedure day sheet
records
relational database
resource utilization groups (RUGs)
schedule of benefits
special purpose applications
superbill
tables
telemedicine
transactions
TRICARE
workers' compensation

REVIEW QUESTIONS

Definitions

Define the following terms:

medical informatics
administrative applications
telemedicine

clinical applications
special purpose applications
bucket billing

Multiple Choice

1. The _____ is a code used by private and government insurers to determine insurance reimbursement.
   A. CPT
   B. DRG
   C. ICD
   D. SWP

2. _____ is defined as the use of technology to organize information in health care.
   A. Computer literacy
   B. Information literacy
   C. Medical informatics
   D. Medical computing

3. The _____ uses of computers include anything that has to do with direct patient care, such as diagnosis, monitoring, and treatment.
   A. Clinical
   B. Administrative
   C. Special purpose
   D. None of the above

4. _____ applications include the use of computers in education and some aspects of pharmacy.
   A. Clinical
   B. Administrative
   C. Special purpose
   D. None of the above

5. _____ applications include the use of computers in office management, scheduling, and planning.
   A. Clinical
   B. Administrative
   C. Special purpose
   D. None of the above

6. Medicare serves _____.
   A. People 65 and over
   B. People with heart conditions
   C. People with chronic renal disorders
   D. A and C

7. A _____ is used to show a patient's outstanding payments.
   A. Patient aging report
   B. Practice analysis report
   C. Patient day sheet
   D. Procedure day sheet

8. A _____ is generated on a monthly basis, and is a summary total of all procedures, charges, and transactions.
   A. Patient aging report
   B. Practice analysis report

    C. Patient day sheet

    D. Procedure day sheet

9. A _____ lists the day's patients, chart numbers, and transactions. It is used for daily reconciliation.

    A. Patient aging report

    B. Practice analysis report

    C. Patient day sheet

    D. Procedure day sheet

10. A _____ is a grouped report organized by procedure.

    A. Patient aging report

    B. Practice analysis report

    C. Payment day sheet

    D. Procedure day sheet

11. A _____ is a grouped report organized by providers.

    A. Patient aging report

    B. Practice analysis report

    C. Payment day sheet

    D. Procedure day sheet

12. Practices that submit electronic claims use a/n _____, a business that collects insurance claims from providers and sends them to the correct insurance carrier.

    A. Insurance collector

    B. Collection agency

    C. Clearinghouse

    D. None of the above

13. The insurance company's response to a paper claim includes a/n _____ which explains why certain services were covered and others not.

    A. Explanation of benefits (EOB)

    B. Electronic remittance advice (ERA)

    C. Lawyer's letter

    D. All of the above

14. The Health Care Financing Administration (HCFA) is now called _____.

    A. Centers for Medicare and Medicaid Services (CMS)

    B. Center for Medical Services (CMS)

    C. Center for Minor Surgery (CMS)

    D. None of the above

15. The insurance company's response to an electronic claim includes a/n _____ which explains why certain services were covered and others not.

    A. Explanation of benefits (EOB)

    B. Electronic remittance advice (ERA)

    C. Lawyer's letter

    D. All of the above

True/False Questions

1. A superbill or encounter form is a list of diagnoses and procedures common to the practice. _____

2. A patient is not responsible for the copayment. _____
3. Charges, payments, and adjustments are called transactions. _____
4. Under fee-for-service insurance plans, the patient is required to pay a deductible before the insurance company will cover medical costs. _____
5. A patient who uses a health maintenance organization (HMO) pays a fixed yearly fee, and can choose among any health care provider or hospital. _____
6. ICD-9-CM provides codes for more than 1,000 diseases. _____
7. Today hospital reimbursement by private and government insurers is determined by diagnosis (DRG). _____
8. Bucket billing is used by medical offices to accommodate two or three insurers, who must be billed in a timely fashion before the patient is billed. _____
9. Doctors who accept assignment require payment by the patient, not the insurance company. _____
10. Encounter form is another term for a patient day sheet. _____

Critical Thinking

1. The computerization of medical records has advantages and disadvantages. Comment on this statement. Do the advantages outweigh the disadvantages? Support your answer.
2. Under our current health care system, some medical decisions are being made by insurance companies. How would you design a system where health care practitioners and patients determined necessary treatments?
3. Comment on how the computerization of administrative tasks may affect a medical office. Bear in mind both efficiency and the fact that an office can print out reports that show the most profitable procedures and practitioners.

SOURCES

Anderson, Sandra. *Computer Literacy for Health Care Professionals.* New York: Delmar Publishers, 1992.

Baase, Sara. *A Gift of Fire: Social, Legal, and Ethical Issues in Computing.* Upper Saddle River, NJ: Prentice-Hall, 1996.

Ball, Marion J., and Kathryn J. Hannah. *Using Computers in Nursing,* Norwalk, CT: Appelton-Century-Crofts, 1984.

Burke, Lillian, and Barbara Weill. *MediSoft Made Easy: A Step-by-Step Approach.* Upper Saddle River, NJ: Prentice-Hall, 2004.

CMS. http://cms.hhs.gov/medicaid/default.asp (September 2002; April 4, 2003).

———. "Medicare Program; Procedures for Coding and Payment Determinations for Clinical Laboratory Tests and for Durable Medical Equipment." http://cms.hhs.gov/medicare/hcpcs/codepayproc.asp (September 25, 2002; February 4, 2004).

Deparle, Nancy-Ann. Testimony on Medicare Payment Reforms before Senate Finance Committee (March 19, 1999; January 13, 2004).

Felton, Bruce. "Technologies That Enable the Disabled." *New York Times,* September 14, 1997.

Gennari, John. http://faculty.washington.edu/gennari/MedicalInformaticsDef.html (July 22, 2002; October 15, 2003).

"Handbook of Medical Informatics." edited by J.H. Van Bemmel and M.A. Musen "American Medical Informatics Association" http://www.mihandbook.standford.edu. (March 23, 1999; May 12, 2004).

Holland, Gina. "Court Backs Regulation of HMOs." *Star-Ledger,* April 3, 2003, p. 43.

Ito, Lloyd. http://phys-advisor.com/Insure.htm (August 3, 1999; October 15, 2003).

Marietti, Charlene. "In Waddles the Solution." Healthcare Informatics Online. www.healthcare-informatics.com (May 2003; May 12, 2004).

"Medical Informatics." http://www.bae.ncsu.edu/bae/research/blanchard/www/465/textbook/otherprojects/1998/infor (1998; March 29, 2003).

OASIS Brochure. http://www.cthomecare.org/OASIS%20Brochure%20-%20CT.pdf (2004; February 7, 2004).

Sanderson, Susan. *Computers in the Medical Office Using MediSoft.* New York: McGraw-Hill, 1995.

Versweyveld, Leslie. "Open Source EMR Programme Can Stimulate Doctors to Embrace Computerisation." *Virtual Medical Worlds Monthly.* http://www.hoise.com/vmw/00/articles/vmw/LV-VM-12-00-8.html (November 6, 2000; January 14, 2004).

Telemedicine

OUTLINE

- Learning Objectives
- Overview
- Store-and-Forward Technology and Interactive Videoconferencing
- Teleradiology
- Telepathology
- Teledermatology
- Telecardiology
- Telestroke
- Telepsychiatry
- Remote Monitoring Devices
- Telehome Care
- Telemedicine in Prison
- Other Uses of Telemedicine
- The Telenurse
- Issues in Telemedicine
- Selected Reading
- Chapter Summary
- Key Terms
- Review Questions
  - *Multiple Choice*
  - *True/False Questions*
  - *Critical Thinking*
- Sources
- Related Web Sites

LEARNING OBJECTIVES

Upon completion of this chapter, you will be able to

- Define telemedicine.
- Describe store-and-forward technology and interactive videoconferencing.

- List the various subspecialties of teleradiology, telepathology, teledermatology, telecardiology, telestroke, telepsychiatry, and telehome care.
- Describe the use of telemedicine in prisons.
- Discuss the changing role of the telenurse.
- Describe the legal, licensing, insurance, and privacy issues involved in telemedicine.

OVERVIEW

Telemedicine uses computers and telecommunications equipment to deliver medical care at a distance. Various technologies are used from plain old telephone service to ISDN lines, to DSL, to dedicated T1 lines, to satellite, to broadband cable, to the Internet. The medical information transmitted can be in any form, including voice, data, still images, and motion video. Telemedicine can deliver the whole range of medical care from diagnosis to patient monitoring to treatment. It gives patients remote access to experts who in turn have access to patient information. The linking of computers and other devices into networks (discussed in chapter 1) forms the foundation for telemedicine. The field of telemedicine is growing at a rapid rate. In 2002, the executive director of the American Telemedicine Association estimated that about 1,000 health care facilities are linked via telecommunications lines. He traces part of this growth to the increased coverage provided by government and private insurers (Jette, 2002). The production of telehome care products grew more quickly in the 1990s than that of any other medical device. There is no comprehensive study of the extent of telemedicine in the United States. However, a study of its use in California concluded that 37 percent of health clinics and one-third of hospitals were using videoconferencing. Telemedicine encompasses many subspecialties of medicine, including radiology, pathology, oncology, ophthalmology, cardiology, stroke, dermatology, and psychiatry. It may involve the sending of still images or real-time conferences, the use of remote monitoring devices, and the remote operation of medical equipment such as microscopes. Varieties of telemedicine are now being used to treat everything from psychiatric disorders (**telepsychiatry**) to skin rashes (**teledermatology**) to cancer (**teleoncology**). Remote surgery is in an early phase and is discussed in a later chapter. The field of telemedicine is changing and developing very rapidly. Telemedicine has the potential of making high-quality medical care available to anyone in an urban or rural area regardless of distance from major medical centers, specialists, physicians, and visiting nurses. It can dramatically decrease the time a patient must wait and the miles he or she must travel to consult a specialist. Telemedicine transfers medical expertise instead of medical experts and patients. Many studies have found that patient satisfaction with telemedicine is high.

Medical consultations and exams at a distance have been attempted from the time that people were able to talk to each other from a distance. Early endeavors were made to send heart and lung sounds to experts over the newly invented telephone. But this failed due to poor transmission. Later, doctors tried to transmit electrocardiograms through the telephone. After World War II, pictures could be transmitted. However, it was only with the development of computers and telecommunications networks capable of transmitting high-resolution digital images and accurate sound that telemedicine could become a practical medical reality. The field is expanding so quickly that it is only possible to touch on major uses of telemedicine here. The following survey introduces the student to basic definitions in the field, and presents examples of some of the more interesting uses of distance medicine. It also discusses some of the technical, legal, privacy, and insurance issues that need to be addressed for telemedicine to fulfill its promise.

STORE-AND-FORWARD TECHNOLOGY AND INTERACTIVE VIDEOCONFERENCING

Telemedicine projects may be based on store-and-forward technology or interactive videoconferencing. Some projects use both. **Store-and-forward technology** involves sharing information in a time- and place-independent way over the Internet. The information is stored, digitized, and then sent. If a medical specialty is image based, store-and-forward technology may be appropriate. The information may include digital images and clinical information. It may be as simple and inexpensive as attaching an image to an e-mail and sending it over phone lines. Store-and-forward technology does not require the sophisticated telecommunications link required by videoconferencing, so it tends to be cheaper. The earliest use of store-and-forward technology was in teleradiology. It is appropriate to specialties where diagnosis is based on images, such as dermatology and pathology. Images can be created by digital camera, and sent over the Internet. For example, this technique is used in some teleopthalmology programs, where others use videoconferencing. Because store-and-forward is cheaper and does not require sophisticated equipment or broadband lines, it is being used simply to introduce telemedicine at low cost to developing countries in specialties that had traditionally used videoconferencing. For example, a small teleneurology program using store-and-forward technology was created between the United Kingdom and Bangladesh. The program was used with 12 patients to deliver expert advice; it was found to be effective.

    Interactive videoconferencing or **teleconferencing** allows doctors to consult with each other and with patients in real time, at a distance. A patient may be in his or her primary physician's office with a camera and a telecommunications link to a specialist's office. Everyone can be seen and heard in real-time. Only a videophone and a connection to the Internet might be required. However, the most sophisticated systems involve microphones, scanners, cameras, medical instruments, and dedicated phone lines. One form of video teleconferencing is the remote house call, involving only one medical practitioner and a patient in another location.

TELERADIOLOGY

The oldest form of telemedicine using computers and telecommunications equipment is teleradiology. Today, teleradiology involves the sending of radiological images in digital form over telecommunications lines. **Teleradiology** uses store-and-forward technology; the data to be sent is digitized, stored, and transmitted over a telecommunications network. If the image is compressed for storage and transmission, and if, as a result, any data is lost, the consultant is responsible for determining if the image is useful. The images can be sent any distance—from across the street to across the world. Store-and-forward teleradiology can be combined with interactive videoconferencing for immediate consultation when a problem is detected in pregnancy. The specialist can see the patient and ultrasound on a split screen and can control the exam from miles away. Before telemedicine, a patient might have to wait for a consultation with a specialist and travel long distances. Now the technology can come to the patient.

TELEPATHOLOGY

Telepathology is the transmission of microscopic images over telecommunications lines. The pathologist sees images on a monitor instead of under a microscope. Telepathology requires a microscope, camera, and monitor, as well as a connection to a telemedicine system. Telepathology can use real-time videoconferencing during an operation for consultation. But in daily practice, store-and-forward is common. Pathology is based on the study of images; diagnosis is based on the study of images on slides from a microscope looking for diagnostic features. If a second opinion is needed from a distant expert, telepathology may be used. The images are taken from the slides by camera. Still images usually are at a higher resolution than those sent in real-time. The images and other clinical data are used for a complete case description, and then sent, in many cases over the Internet. One of the problems of store-and-forward telepathology is the choice of images sent. They may not show a complete picture, and this may lead to misdiagnosis.

TELEDERMATOLOGY

Teledermatology (the practice of dermatology using telecommunications networks) is also based partly on the study of images. It uses both videoconferencing and store-and-forward technology. Both methods appear effective. The advantage of the videoconference is that it closely resembles the traditional visit to the doctor, but is more expensive. Studies have shown that diagnosis made via videoconferencing agree with face-to-face dermatology visits 59 to 88 percent of the time. A small study comparing store-and-forward teledermatology with face-to-face dermatology found a 61 to 91 percent agreement. Certain skin conditions were found to be more difficult to diagnose via teledermatology. Diagnostic confidence was lower and the rate of biopsies higher. The advantage of store-and-forward is the high quality of the images and the low cost. To date there have been no definitive outcomes studies. Some small studies have found that although there are limitations with store-and-forward (image quality and lack of patient interaction), teledermatology reduced unnecessary visits to dermatologists by more than 50 percent. A small pilot study found that teledermatology was useful at assessing skin conditions (Dupree, 2003).

TELECARDIOLOGY

Prior to the 1800s, a doctor would listen to the heart by placing his ear on the patient's chest. Listening to the heart at a distance has a long history.

> In 1816, Dr. Rene Laennec, an expert in chest diseases, was examining a young woman with heart problems. Painfully shy, he could not bring himself to press his ear to her chest. . . . he made a "log" by rolling sheets of paper into a cylinder. Laennec recalled applying one end of it to the region of the heart and the other to his ear, and was surprised to find that he could perceive the action of the heart in a manner much more clear and distinct. "The American Experience: Gallery: Medical Instruments and Teaching Aids." http://www.pbs.org/wgbh/amex/murder/gallery/g_13 (2003; October 7, 2003)

Since the invention of the telephone, doctors have attempted to send heart and lung sounds over long distances. But the quality of the sound was not good enough. During the 1960s, it became possible to transmit heart sounds more accurately, and faxes can be used to send EKGs. By the 1990s echocardiograms could be telecommunicated. Second opinions via telecardiology are one of the most common requests in telemedicine. People come into rural emergency rooms with chest pains, and many ER doctors want an expert consultation. Telemedicine is becoming more and more widely used in cardiology. One study evaluated five programs in North America: two use store-and-forward and three use real-time. The study concluded that real-time and store-and-forward tele-echocardiography are effective; both transmit diagnostic-quality information.

Other telecommunications technology contributes to cardiac care. The Department of Veterans' Affairs will be able to use an Internet-based service that connects patients wearing pacemakers with their doctors. Patients will be able to use a monitoring device to collect information from the pacemaker by holding an antenna over it. The data is sent by phone to the CareLink Network. Doctors can then have access to it. This system will work anywhere in the United States. Another technology that can be used to connect digital devices is **Bluetooth**. Bluetooth technology can link devices such as a pacemaker and a cell phone. When the pacemaker senses a dangerous event, the cell phone automatically calls 911.

TELESTROKE

One of the recognized benefits of telemedicine is saving time. This is essential in treating strokes. There are almost three-quarters of a million new strokes per year in the United States. If the stroke is caused by a clot (determined by a CT scan), the victim may be helped by the administration of a clot-busting drug called t-PA if it is given within a few hours. However, if the stroke is caused by excessive bleeding, t-PA can kill the patient. Immediate and accurate diagnosis is crucial. However, many small hospitals do not have experts. One study showed that 70 percent of stroke patients did not receive t-PA either because they arrived at the hospital too late or because the hospitals could not provide the correct therapy. Massachusetts General Hospital began a **telestroke** program. Many people die of strokes just because they are taken to small hospitals without the capability of evaluating the stroke quickly. The telestroke program connects small local hospitals with Massachusetts General's stroke experts. When a stroke victim appeared at a local hospital in Martha's Vineyard, the doctors would do CT scans, then forward them to stroke specialists at Mass General. Both the local doctors and the specialists would evaluate the tests and interview the patient via a teleconferencing system to determine whether t-PA was needed. Other hospitals are currently using this technology. The federal Stop Stroke Act, which has not yet become law, would provide funding to build telestroke systems.

TELEPSYCHIATRY

Telepsychiatry involves the delivery of therapy using teleconferencing. It usually makes use of some sort of hardware that can transmit and receive both voice and picture. However, in order to cut costs, psychiatrists are trying to find out if a poor image— or no image at all—makes therapy less effective. Experts warn that therapy at a distance is not a substitute for the human contact involved in face-to-face counseling. However, sometimes it is the only choice, for example, in rural areas where there are very few therapists and patients would have to travel long distances to see them.

During the 1960s, the first telepsychiatry sessions were conducted at the Nebraska Psychiatric Institute. Researchers found that the fact that the therapist was not physically present had little effect on group therapy. Studies of psychiatric consults between primary care providers and psychiatrists in New Hampshire came to the same conclusion—that videoconferencing and face-to-face consults were similar. A study of telemedicine for diagnosing patients with obsessive-compulsive disorder found it as successful as face-to-face therapy. A small study compared videoconferencing and face-to-face cognitive behavioral therapy in treating childhood depression and found them equally effective (Nelson, 2003). Some studies have found patients more comfortable talking to a distant psychiatrist. Others found that using a telenurse and a traditional psychiatrist improved depression more than simply a psychiatrist, although there was no improvement in the numbers of clients taking their medication properly. Telepsychiatry was also found to be successful in delivering therapy to the family of a girl suffering from anorexia. It contributed to her recovery. The family was satisfied with the teletherapy (Goldfield and Boachie, 2003). However, there are some negative aspects to telepsychiatry. The technology limits the therapist's perception of nonverbal clues, and the equipment can be distracting. The therapist has to be sensitive to distortions in eye contact and the fact that a patient can appear to have stopped speaking when in fact he or she has not, that is, eye contact must be maintained with the camera, not the monitor and the patient's mouth may stop moving before the patient has stopped speaking. One 18-month study of telepsychiatry in a prison setting found that patients were comfortable with the technology, but that many of the therapist's recommendations were not followed by prison personnel. This was a unique situation. The psychiatrist did not have some of the clients' medical records and so some recommendations (e.g., that a woman in a wheelchair ride a bike) could not be carried out. Other recommendations were not carried out either because the doctor had little knowledge of prison rules and routines or the doctor had no relationship with prison personnel. The psychiatrist had never been to the prison, and the medical records (which were paper records) had to stay at the prison. This points out some of the limitations of telepsychiatry—clues that would be easily available in person are not obvious via telecommunications lines (Turner, 2001).

There are questions of whether telepsychiatry is appropriate for some forms of serious mental illness. For example, can schizophrenia be made worse by reinforcing the delusion that the television is talking to the patient?

REMOTE MONITORING DEVICES

Remote monitoring devices make it possible for patients to be monitored at home. A **telespirometry** system can be used at home by asthmatic patients; it is designed to transmit over the telephone to a remote location. A portable fetal monitor allows test results to be transmitted to a remote location. A miniature ECG Telemetry system allows wireless remote **arrhythmia monitoring**. Remote monitoring devices are also used in ambulances. The condition of the patient can be directly transmitted to the emergency room so that care can begin immediately on arrival. In September 1998, a "smart stretcher" was introduced. Weighing 135 pounds, but only 5 inches high, the stretcher includes a respirator, heart machine, intravenous drugs, and monitors that transmit all the data they gather immediately to the hospital. Using the smart stretcher means that no time needs to be wasted transporting the patient. Monitoring and treatment can begin immediately. The Defense Advanced Research Projects Agency of the U.S. Defense Department has created a smart T-shirt that can monitor vital signs at a distance. Distance monitoring of blood-glucose levels have improved outcomes in diabetes patients. In 2002, the FDA approved an implantable cardiac device that enables a doctor to evaluate a patient over the Internet. Not all distance monitoring is successful, however. Distance monitoring of high-risk pregnancies has been a failure (Lewis, 2001).

TELEHOME CARE

Telehome care involves the monitoring of vital signs from a distance via telecommunications equipment and the replacement of home nursing visits with videoconferences. It is usually used to manage chronic conditions such as congestive heart failure and diabetes, but it should be noted that it is beginning to be used for remote monitoring by ICU doctors at home. The cost of medical care for chronic conditions is about 75 percent of U.S. medical costs, and some believe that home monitoring can lower these costs. The number of insurers that cover home monitoring is up from three in 2000, to 20 at the end of 2002. Some large hospitals have received grants from the Centers for Medicare and Medicaid Services (CMS) to expand telehome care. Some of this money will be used for demonstration projects and randomized trials.

Telehome care involves a link between the patient's home and a hospital or central office that collects the data. Equipment ($2,000–$6,000 per unit) is installed in the patient's home. It links the home via telecommunications lines with a central office. The units differ from one another, but generally allow the patient and nurse to see and hear each other. The patient can push a button on the monitor, enabling the nurse to hear heart, lung, and bowel sounds; another button allows the nurse to monitor blood pressure. The machines also assess blood-oxygen level and pulse rate. Many units give voice reminders to take medication, and ask the patient questions. HANC (home assisted nursing care), for example, yells more and more loudly until the patient responds. Some of the programs include extensive education about home management of chronic illness and even provide a tele–social worker for end-of-life planning. There have not been any large-scale randomized studies of telehome care. Pilot studies have indicated that telehome care does increase access to health care in rural areas, and that it may decrease unnecessary hospital and emergency room visits. It allows a nurse to make many more visits in a day—15 to 20 instead of 5 to 6. A small United States–United Kingdom study concluded that 45 percent of U.S. home visits could be remote. Many small studies have found both nurses and patients like the video visits, and one study found that telehospice care was quite cost effective. A study in Italy found home telemonitoring for patients with severe respiratory illness decreased hospital admissions, and patients were satisfied. The study concluded that telemonitoring can provide high-quality home care (Maiolo et al., 2003). Another small study found telemedicine effective in reducing hospital admissions for patients with congestive heart failure; patients had their vital signs and general appearance telemonitored while maintaining regular video contact with health care professionals who offered advice on drug use and diet. In California, a study compared the use of face-to-face with videoconferencing in control and intervention groups. No differences in medication compliance, knowledge of disease, and ability for self-care were found. Patients were satisfied with the videoconferencing. Further, it costs less to treat patients via teleconferencing than face-to-face (Johnson et al., 2000). Several factors prevent the adoption of telehome care, including the attitudes of home health agencies, the initial cost of the equipment, reimbursement rates, and the lack of studies demonstrating that it is cost effective.

TELEMEDICINE IN PRISON

Telemedicine is now widely used in state prisons in Arizona, Iowa, Maryland, Texas, Massachusetts, Virginia, Pennsylvania, and New York, and in the federal prison system. The stated reasons for introducing telemedicine are cost containment, security, and enhanced medical care for inmates. Telemedicine is used to provide specialist care, not primary care, which is delivered on-site. Although no comprehensive study exists, there are some comparisons of traditional to telemedical care in specific areas. The Arizona Department of Corrections did a cost-benefit analysis in FY 2000 and found a $200.89 savings per case, which came to a total savings of $156,694.20. A review of the literature on Texas indicates that both patients and providers are satisfied with the care and that the vast majority of systems experienced reductions in travel and security costs. One preliminary study found that 95 percent of the telemedical consults have saved a trip to a clinic. A teleconsult clinic for HIV positive inmates was established in Texas in 1999: it was found to cut costs, but have no effect on outcomes. Massachusetts also introduced a telemedicine program for HIV positive prisoners and found no significant differences in health outcomes. However, HIV patients became increasingly concerned about privacy. Further study of this project is planned. There seems to be a consensus that telemedicine in prisons saves money and increases security by decreasing off-site visits. Survey data also indicates that both prisoners and prison administrators are satisfied with telemedicine. It may be that more prisoners seek treatment because they do not have to travel. In states such as Texas, a visit to a clinic can mean four days of travel shackled in a truck. However, there are no comprehensive studies on the effect on the health of prisoners.

OTHER USES OF TELEMEDICINE

In 1996, the federal government funded 19 pilot projects in telemedicine. Many are now taken-for-granted aspects of telemedicine: attempts to bring health care to rural areas and attempts to link small hospitals with medical centers for sharing of information. Others sent medication reminders to the elderly. One tested an adverse drug event monitor. These programs are now in common use and are discussed in the chapter on pharmacy. One of the more interesting and highly successful programs is **Baby CareLink**. Baby CareLink was originated in Massachusetts. Its purpose was to compare high-risk, premature infants receiving traditional care with an experimental group, which, in addition to traditional care, received a telemedicine link to the hospital while the babies were hospitalized and for six months after. The families could see and hear their babies in the nursery even though they were at home. They could log on to a secure Web page with up-to-date information about their babies. Once home, the families had access to the nursery and experts and could ask any question they pleased. The doctor or nurse could see the baby and reassure the parent. One purpose of Baby CareLink was to see if parents felt more comfortable and knowledgeable about their babies' care, so that the hospital stay would be shorter. The experimental group did have shorter hospital stays. In a later case study of Baby CareLink in Chicago, it was found that the average length of stay for the experimental group was 2.73 days shorter, that only 18 percent were readmitted (less than the expected 40 percent), medical staff were happy with the program, and parents were more comfortable with their infants. Baby CareLink is now covered by several state Medicaid programs and at least one private insurer. Baby CareLink is currently established in many hospitals throughout the country.

In Texas and Kansas, day care centers have brought teledoctors to day care. An on-site nurse uses a video camera and stethoscope and other equipment. A doctor diagnoses the child. In the vast majority of cases, the child is allowed to stay at day care, and a prescription is called in. The parent does not have to leave work. In Rochester, New York, a federal grant is helping to set up a telemedicine system serving day care centers.

Telemedicine is currently being utilized in almost every aspect of health care. One of the more interesting new uses of telemedicine is in Vermont in a tele-trauma project that links trauma surgeon's homes with hospital emergency departments, providing immediate expert service at any time (Ricci, 2003).

Telemedicine is being used in weight management and pain management. Teleoncology systems are helping cancer patients avoid lengthy trips to the doctor and feel more secure because they have a 24-hour link to health care.

In hospitals and even operating rooms, health care personnel (including 17 percent of doctors) are making use of personal digital assistants for writing prescriptions, quickly accessing patient information, and finding facts in online databases of medical articles and journals.

THE TELENURSE

Telemedicine is changing the role of the nurse. **Telenursing** involves both teletriage and the telecommunication of health-related data, the remote house call, and the monitoring of chronic disease. **Teletriage** starts with a call from a worried patient or parent with a question to the nurse. Software helps the nurse ask a series of questions to aid in diagnosis and make a recommendation to the patient. Telenursing increases access to medical advice by making it available in their homes. Nurses may be in more autonomous positions in telemedicine programs. In England there is a 24-hour phone line staffed by nurses. The nurses use diagnostic software and are linked to databases, hospitals, primary care providers, and ambulances. The nurses staffing these lines need to know how to use the software and how to get correct information; she or he also needs knowledge of local health care services. In the United States, the Veterans Affairs telephone care program is staffed by RNs only. The nurses have access to the patient records and to the primary care provider through e-mail. Patients appreciate the immediate attention from an expert.

In teleconferencing the nurse takes the patient's vital signs from a distance and assesses the patient via a monitor. Although the televisit is similar to the actual visit, it is not identical. Nurses lead many telemedicine programs. In some programs nurses perform diagnostic services. Nurses need to be familiar with computerized equipment and comfortable using it. When telemedicine is used in schools, the school nurse becomes responsible for the referral and follows up on home care. Nurses involved in a study of the role of telehealth in psychiatry needed knowledge of management of depression, medication, counseling, and the ability to provide emotional support. In a telemedicine project examining diabetes, the nurse case manager performed weekly consultations, and the doctor monthly consultations. The nurse would recommend changes in diet and exercise and participate in the doctor's monthly consult.

ISSUES IN TELEMEDICINE

For telemedicine to fulfill its promise, certain technical, legal, insurance, and privacy issues need to be addressed. On the technical side, an appropriate telecommunications infrastructure must be in place. The Telecommunications Act of 1996 proposes that access be increased, but does not specify how. Certain aspects of telemedicine require high-speed, broadband media, since the files transmitted may be so huge (greater than 1 gigabyte). This applies particularly to the utilization of real-time interactive video teleconferencing, which transmits voice, sound, images, text, and motion video.

In addition, legal issues such as licensing, medical liability, and privacy concerns need to be addressed. Furthermore, there are problems of insurance. Currently, there is minimal insurance coverage for telemedicine, although this is changing slowly. If the Medicare Remote Monitoring Services Coverage Act becomes law, Medicare would cover the remote house call. Currently Medicare and most private insurers cover only face-to-face medical care, with exceptions. As of January 1, 1999, the Balanced Budget Act of 1997 required that Medicare pay for telemedical services in medically underserved areas. However, after two years of this expanded reimbursement, Medicare had only reimbursed $20,000 for 301 teleconsultation claims. In an attempt to expand coverage further, Congress passed the Medicare, Medicaid, and SCHIP Benefits Improvement and Protection Act. It went into effect in October 2001. Twenty state Medicaid programs now cover some telemedicine services, as do some private insurers. In California, Texas, and Louisiana, it is illegal for insurers to discriminate between face-to-face and telemedical services.

One of the most serious legal obstacles to the development of telemedicine is state licensing. Medical personnel are required to be licensed by the state in which they practice. Acquiring a license is a costly and time-consuming process. Practicing without a license is a crime. Licensing laws are different in each state. Some states allow consultations across state lines. However, the American Medical Association supports requiring physicians to be licensed in any state in which they practice telemedicine. Some states have reciprocity agreements with other states. Between 1997 and 2001, the number of states adopting laws on the practice of telemedicine rose from 11 to 26; many of these laws are restrictive and require telemedicine providers to be separately licensed in each jurisdiction. Only 12 states have agreements that make it easier for nurses to practice across state lines.

Telemedicine raises many privacy issues. Medical information routinely crosses state lines, some of it via e-mail, which is not private. There are typically nonmedical personnel involved, including technicians and camera operators. According to the Final HIPAA Privacy Rules, several privacy issues are relevant. Under HIPAA, "Federal laws preempt state laws that are in conflict with regulatory requirements or those that provide less stringent privacy protections. But those states that have *more* stringent privacy laws would preempt Federal law." This leads to a "patchwork" of different standards. In a telemedical consultation, many people (both medical and nonmedical) may be present—but are not apparent to the patient. Telemedicine requires greater concern with patient privacy and more complicated consent from patients.

The laws concerning telemedicine today are ambiguous; legal liability is not clear. It is not even clear what pieces of equipment used in a telemedical consult or exam are considered medical devices and are therefore subject to regulation by the Food and Drug Administration. Some of the legal ramifications are made clear by the following hypothetical cases:

- "A public figure is hospitalized with a mental illness. Upon her release, she consults with her psychiatrist by telephone. These conversations and her medical records are stored in a computer database. A reporter 'hacks' his way into these records and prints a story containing damaging information. *Who is liable?*" (Emphasis added.)
- "A family practitioner in Virginia sees an unusual spot on an X-ray. She transmits the image to a radiologist in Pennsylvania who misreads the X-ray, resulting in a misdiagnosis. The patient, who lives in Maryland, dies. *When the patient's family brings suit in Maryland, are the practitioners subject to jurisdiction in that state and which state's medical malpractice law will apply?*" (Emphasis added.)

The answers to these questions are not yet clear.

SELECTED READING

John O'Neil. "Telemedicine, the Easy Way." *New York Times,* October 1, 2002.

IN THE NEWS

Vital Signs: Techniques; Telemedicine, the Easy Way

by John O'Neil

Telemedicine can be successful without being complicated, Australian doctors said in a case report being published today.

It describes a mother's makeshift system that allowed her son to complete his recovery from burns at their rural home rather than in a specialized hospital hundreds of miles away.

The report, in *The Journal of Telemedicine and Telecare,* concerns a 14-year-old boy from Queensland who required a skin graft after he burned his leg with the exhaust from his motorcycle.

When his doctors and nurses noticed signs of deterioration of the skin graft before he was to be discharged from the Royal Children's Hospital in Brisbane, members of the team in charge of his care considered extending his stay.

But then, the mother of the boy came up with a plan that allowed him to return home, according to Anthony Smith of the University of Queensland's online health center.

The mother used a digital scanner, which converts printed material into computer files, to take pictures of her son's leg by having him place it on top of the scanner—just as an office prankster would use a copying machine to take a picture of his face by scrunching it against the glass.

The mother sent the images to the Brisbane hospital by e-mail every other day for 8 weeks, then once a week for an additional 12 weeks.

(continued)

The mother talked regularly to members of the burn unit team by telephone. And, once every few weeks, a meeting was held by videoconference between the burn specialists in Brisbane and the physicians at the regional hospital nearest the boy.

October 1, 2002. Copyright © 2002 by The New York Times Company. Reprinted by permission.

CHAPTER SUMMARY

Chapter 4 introduces the reader to the field of telemedicine and some of its subspecialties. In addition, its effectiveness and some of the issues that must be addressed for telemedicine to fully develop are discussed.

- Telemedicine uses computers and telecommunications technology to deliver health care, including diagnosis, patient monitoring, and treatment at a distance. As such, it has the potential of making high-quality health care available to anyone regardless of distance from major medical centers. It may use store-and-forward technology for transmission of still images or interactive videoconferencing for real-time consultations.
- It encompasses subspecialties such as teleradiology, telepathology, telecardiology, telestroke, telehome care, and telepsychiatry, as well as the use of remote monitoring devices and remote operation of medical equipment.
- Remote monitoring devices allow patients to be monitored at home or in an ambulance. The information is transmitted to a remote location.
- Telemedicine is changing the role of the nurse.
- Telemedicine is currently being evaluated, and the assessments tend to be positive. It is used in prison settings where its efficacy is being judged. Several studies have been completed and more are underway. The federal government has funded several projects to be evaluated.
- For the promise of telemedicine to be fulfilled, certain problems have to be solved. These include the establishment of adequate high bandwidth communications lines, barriers posed by state licensing, the lack of insurance coverage, and the insecurity of the electronic medical record. HIPAA addresses some of the privacy problems posed by telemedicine.

KEY TERMS

arrhythmia monitoring
Baby CareLink
Bluetooth
interactive video-
  conferencing

remote monitoring
  devices
store-and-forward
  technology
teleconferencing

teledermatology
telehome care
telemedicine
telenursing
teleoncology

telepathology   teleradiology   telestroke
telepsychiatry   telespirometry   teletriage

REVIEW QUESTIONS

Multiple Choice

1. Telemedicine involves _____.
   A. The linking of doctors and patients at a distance
   B. The transmission of radiologic images via telecommunications lines
   C. The transmission of patient data in any form
   D. All of the above
2. The technology used in teleradiology is called _____.
   A. Send-and-receive
   B. Receive-and-send
   C. Store-and-forward
   D. None of the above
3. Before telemedicine can deliver high-quality medical services at a distance _____.
   A. A reliable broadband telecommunications network has to be in place
   B. State licensing barriers have to be overcome
   C. Every patient needs to own a printer
   D. A and B only
4. The transmission of microscopic images over telecommunications lines is called _____.
   A. Teleradiology
   B. Telepsychiatry
   C. Telepathology
   D. Remote monitoring
5. Telemedicine projects in prisons have been found to _____.
   A. Improve health care
   B. Cut costs
   C. Improve security
   D. All of the above
6. _____ allows doctors and patients to consult in real time, at a distance.
   A. Telepathology
   B. Teleradiology
   C. Teleoncology
   D. Interactive videoconferencing
7. Which of the following is true about telemedicine?
   A. It is used to treat depression.
   B. It delivers medical care to prisoners.
   C. It can deliver the whole range of medical care from diagnosis to treatment.
   D. All of the above.

8. Telemedicine is used in some way in the treatment of _____.
   A. Psychiatric disorders
   B. Cancer
   C. Skin rashes
   D. All of the above
9. Remote medical consultations and exams were first tried _____.
   A. After World War II
   B. In 1997
   C. As soon as the telephone was invented
   D. In 1977
10. A remote house call by a visiting nurse is an example of _____.
    A. Telepathology
    B. Teleradiology
    C. Video teleconferencing
    D. None of the above
11. _____ technology is used to link electronic devices (e.g., a pacemaker with a cell phone).
    A. Telephone
    B. Bluetooth
    C. Video teleconferencing
    D. Store-and-forward
12. The _____ program at Massachusetts General Hospital diagnoses quickly and can determine if t-PA should be used in treatment.
    A. Telestroke
    B. Telecardiology
    C. Telenurse
    D. Teledoctor
13. One of the most successful telemedicine programs links hospitalized premature infants with their parents at home. It is called _____.
    A. TeleBaby
    B. Computer Parenting
    C. TelePreemie
    D. Baby CareLink
14. Many telemedicine programs have been found to be effective. But _____ is not.
    A. Distance monitoring of problem pregnancies
    B. Telehome care
    C. Telemedicine in prisons
    D. Teletriage programs run by telenurses
15. In Vermont a _____ project links trauma surgeons' homes with hospital emergency departments.
    A. Telestroke
    B. Tele-trauma
    C. Telecardiology
    D. Teleoncology

True/False Questions

1. Most medical insurance now covers telemedicine as well as face-to-face medicine. ____F____
2. The broadband links are in place to deliver telemedicine all over the world. ____T____
3. State licensing of doctors is an obstacle to the development of telemedicine. ____T____
4. The electronic patient record is absolutely secure. ____F____
5. The oldest form of telemedicine is teleradiology. ____T____
6. Telemedicine has the potential of giving immediate access to specialists regardless of distance. ____T____
7. In a telemedical consult, many people (both medical and nonmedical) may be present. ____F____
8. Telepsychiatry is recommended therapy for anyone regardless of mental disorder. ____F____
9. By the 1990s echocardiograms could be telecommunicated. ____T____
10. Remote monitoring devices make it possible for patients to be monitored at home. ____T____

Critical Thinking

1. Cite some examples of the current usage of aspects of telemedicine technologies in the diagnosis and treatment of patients. Can you suggest future uses of telemedicine that would improve health care?
2. How can patient confidentiality be safeguarded, given the insecurity of electronic medical information crossing state lines?
3. Discuss who should be held accountable for mistakes in diagnosis and treatment when there are several parties involved, including the on-site physician, remote specialist and other medical personnel, telecommunications equipment manufacturer, and so on.
4. Should medical personnel involved in telemedicine be licensed in every state or licensed nationally? Discuss the advantages and disadvantages of each.
5. Today, medical personnel need to be retrained in certain telemedicine technology areas. How would you convince them to retrain?

SOURCES

Ace, Allen, Dave Ermer, Gary Doolittle, Pamela Whitten, and Charles Zaylor. "Telemedicine in Kansas: Beyond Anecdotes," American Telemedicine Association Annual Conference Index of 1997 Conference Abstracts. http://www.americantelemed.org/conf/abk.html (1997; October 9, 2003).

"American Experience: Gallery: Medical Instruments and Teaching Aids, The." http://www.pbs.org/wgbh/amex/murder/gallery/g_13 (2003; October 7, 2003).

American Heart Association. "Stroke Treatment and Ongoing Prevention Act: Fact Sheet." Americanheart.org (May 25, 2003; May 25, 2003).

American Indian Diabetic Teleopthalmology Grant Program. abc.hsc.usc.edu/aidr (n.d.; March 18, 2003).

Austen, Ian. "Palmtops in the Operating Room." nyt.com (August 22, 2002; August 22, 2002).

Baby CareLink in the News. "Clinician Support Technology Announces Major Enhancements in 2003 Release of Baby CareLink." http://www.babycarelink.com/news (April 1, 2003; October 13, 2003).

———. "Clinician Support Technology Helps Colorado Develop New Infant Care Program for Hospitals." http://www.babycarelink.com/news (2002; May 17, 2003).

———. "Iowa Hospitals to Use CST's Baby CareLink to Improve Care of Premature Infants." http://www.babycarelink.com/news (December 3, 2002; May 17, 2003).

———. "Medicaid Case Study: Mount Sinai Hospital in Chicago." http://www.babycarelink.com/news (2002; May 17, 2003).

———. "More Than a Baby Monitor." CBS News. http://www.babycarelink.com/news (2002; March 9, 2003).

Bates, James, Barbara R. Demuth, Christine M. Trimbath, Bonnie Pepon, Seong K. Mun, and Betty Levine. "Telemedicine versus Traditional Therapy in the Management of Diabetes" (Abstract). *Telemedicine Journal and e-Health.* tie.telemed.org (April 2003; May 24, 2003).

Beth Israel Deaconess Medical Center Baby CareLink. "Welcome to the NICU." Harvard.edu (1998; November 8, 2000).

Brown, Nancy, and Robert Roberts. "Telemedicine Information Exchange News." tie.telemed.org (March 5, 2003; May 2003).

Burg, Gunter. "Store-and-Forward Teledermatology." emedicine.com (July 17, 2002; May 14, 2003).

Burnett, Lee. "Pocket Computers." *HIPPOCRATES* 14 no. 8 (August 2000). hippocrates.com (August 2000; August 14, 2003).

Chin, Tyler. "Remote Monitoring: The Growth of Home Monitoring." amednews.com (November 18, 2002; May 27, 2003).

"Components of a Telepathology System." Fletcher Allen Health Care. http://www.vtmednet.org/telemedicine/path.htm, pp. 1–2 (December 15, 1998; October 7, 2003).

"Comprehensive Telehealth Act of 1997, The." Arent Fox. http://www.arentfox.com/telemed/federal//bills/97/s385_97.html, pp. 1–2 (1997; May 29, 1999).

"Computers Broaden Capabilities in Medicine." *Doctor's Guide Medical and Other News,* http://www.pslgroup.com/ dg/2CB4A.htm, p. 1 (June 18, 1997; May 29, 1999).

"Conrad Introduces Telehealth Bill." Press release, http://www.arentfox.com/telemed/federal/pressrelease/senconrad0397.html, pp. 1–2 (May 3, 1997; May 29, 1999).

Dakins, Deborah R. "Telemedicine Evaluation Efforts Come into Focus." *Telemedicine* (December 1, 1996). http://www.telemedmag.com/db_archives/1996/961201n1.htm. p. 1 (1997; May 29, 1999).

Dobbin, Ben. "Day Care Center for Low-Income Families Gets a Telemedicine Portal." stopgettingsick.com (May 25, 2003; May 28, 2003).

Doolittle, G. C. "Pilot Data from an Efficacy Study in Teleoncology Practice." American Telemedicine Association Annual Conference Index of 1997 Conference Abstracts. http://www.americantelemedicine.org (1997; October 11, 2003).

Doolittle, G. C., A.R. Williams, and D.J. Cook. "An Estimation of Costs of a Pediatric Telemedicine practice in Public Schools" (Abstract). www.ncbi.nlm.nih.gov (January 2004; October 11, 2003).

"Dramatic Consultations Using Telemedicine: Telemedicine Success Stories." http://telehealth.hrsa.gov/success (December 2000; October 8, 2003).

Dupree, N. E., A. Moshell, M. Turner, G. Del Rosso, J. Kvedar, A. A. Qureshi, and J.L. Ternullo. "Digital Images to Assess Skin Conditions in the US Population" (Abstract). *Telemedicine Journal and e-Health,* 9 (suppl. 1): S1–S37. tie.telemed.org (2003; May 24, 2003).

Federal Telemedicine Legislation 105th Congress, Arent Fox. http://www.crecre.com (n.d.; October 9, 2003).

Federal Telemedicine Update. Federal Telemedicine News. Telemedicine.com (January 22, 2002; October 13, 2003).

————. Federal Telemedicine News. Telemedicine.com (August 15, 2002; May 27, 2003).

————. Federal Telemedicine News. Telemedicine.com (August 19, 2002; October 13, 2003).

Fischman, Josh. "Bringing Doctors to Day Care." usnews.com (May 27, 2002; May 28, 2003).

Garshnek, V., J.S. Logan, and L.H. Hassell. "The Telemedicine Frontier: Going the Extra Mile." www.quasar.org (no date; October 9, 2003).

Goldfield, G. S., and A. Boachie. "Delivery of Family Therapy in the Treatment of Anorexia Nervosa Using Telehealth: A Case Report" (Abstract). *Telemedicine Journal and e-Health* 9 no. 1 (Spring 2003): 111–14. tie.telemed.org (2003; April 16, 2003).

"Great-West Insurer First Commercial User of CST's Baby CareLink Neonatal Care Programme." *Virtual Medical Worlds Monthly.* hoise.com (October 21, 2002; May 17, 2003).

Hafner, Katie. "Why Doctors Don't E-mail." nyt.com (June 6, 2002; August 30, 2002).

Hoffmann, Allan. "Is There a Doctor in the Net?" *Star-Ledger,* April 6, 1998, pp. 21, 25.

Introduction to Telemedicine. *Telemedicine Today.* www2.telemedtoday.com/about.shtml (2002; May 14, 2003).

Jette, Julie. "A Life-Saving Link: Stroke Patients Can Connect with Mass General." neuro-oas .mgh.Harvard.edu/stopstroke/Ledger_5_16_02/htm (May 16, 2002; May 14, 2003).

Johnston, B., L. Wheeler, J. Deuser, and K.H. Sousa. "Outcomes of the Kaiser Permanente Tele-Home Health Research Project" (Abstract). tie.telemed.org (January 2000; October 13, 2003).

Kincaid, Kathy. "Telemedicine Passes Accuracy Test for Cardiology." *Telemedicine* (April 1998): 2.

Kloss-Thompson, Kathy. "Telemedicine and the Congestive Heart Failure Patient" (Abstract). *Telemedicine Journal and e-Health* 9 (Suppl. 1): S1–S29. tie.telemed.org (2003; May 24, 2003).

Laino, Charlene. "Virtual Medicine, Real Benefits." MSNBC, May 28, 1998. http://www.msnbc.com/news/ 168944.asp, pp. 1–6 (May 28, 1998; May 29, 1999).

Landa, Amy Snow. "Telemedicine Expansion Sought." amednews.com (July 15, 2002; May 17, 2003).

Lesher, Jack L. Jr., L.S. Davis, F.W. Gourdin, D. English, and W.O. Thompson. "Telemedicine Evaluation of Cutaneous Diseases: A Blinded Comparative Study" (Abstract). *Journal of the American Academy of Dermatology* 38 no. 1 (January 1998). www.ncbi.nlm.nih.gov (January 1998; October 10, 2003).

Lewis, Carol. "Emerging Trends in Medical Device Technology: Home Is Where the Heart Monitor Is." *FDA Consumer.* FDA.gov (May–June 2001; May 27, 2003).

"Literature Review on Aspects of Nursing Education: The Types of Skills and Knowledge Required to Meet the Changing Needs of the Labour Force Involved in Nursing." dest.gov.au (December 14, 2001; May 17, 2003).

Maddox, Peggy Jo. "Ethics and the Brave New World of E-Health." http://www.nursingworld.org (November 21, 2002; March 18, 2003).

Maiolo, Carmela, Ehab I. Mohamed, Cesare M. Fiorani, and Antonio de Lorenzo. "Home Telemonitoring for Patients with Severe Respiratory Illness: The Italian Experience" (Abstract). *Journal of Telemedicine and Telecare* 9 no. 2 (April 2003): 67–71. www.ncbi.nlm.nih.gov (April 9, 2003; May 24, 2003).

Mea, Vincenzo Della. "Store-and-Forward Telepathology." telemed.uniud.it (1999; October 11, 2003).

Montana Office of Rural Health. "Rural Community-Based Home Health Care and Support Services—A White Paper." healthinfo.montana.edu (August 2001; May 17, 2003).

Murphy, Kate. "Telemedicine Getting a Test in Efforts to Cut Costs of Treating Prisoners." *New York Times,* June 8, 1998, p. D5.

Nelson, E.L., M. Barnard, and S. Cain. "Treating Childhood Depression over Videoconferencing" (Abstract). *Telemedicine Journal and E-Health* 9 no. 1 (Spring 2003): 49–55. tie.telemed.org (2003; April 16, 2003).

NLM National Telemedicine Initiative. Summaries of Awards, October 1996. http://www.nlm.gov/research/initprojsum.html, pp. 1–2 (October 1996; May 29, 1999).

Nucci, Peter. U.S. Department of Justice Office of Justice Programs. National Institute of Justice. "Telemedicine." http://www.ncjrs.org/telemedicine (March 1999; October 10, 2003).

Office of Telemedicine. Department of Corrections, Virginia. Virginia.edu (n.d.; May 17, 2003).

Ohio Department of Rehabilitation and Correction Technology. Telemedicine drc.state.oh.us (January 8, 2001; May 17, 2003).

Paar, David. "Telemedicine in Practice: Texas Department of Criminal Justice." UTMB Correctional Managed Care. utmb.edu (May 2000; May 17, 2003).

Pak, H.S. "A Teledermatology Outcomes Study: A Prospective Randomized Evaluation" (Abstract). *Telemedicine Journal and E-Health* 9 (Suppl 1): 37. tie.telemed.org (April 2003; May 24, 2003).

Patterson, Victor, Fazlul Hoque, David Vassallo, Mike Farquharson Roberts, Pat Swinfen, and Roger Swinfen. "Store-and-Forward Teleneurology in Developing Countries." *Journal of Telemedicine and Telecare* 7 (Suppl. 1): 52–53 www.coh.uq.edu.au (2001; October 13, 2003).

Raimer, Ben, Patti Patterson, and Oscar Boultinghouse. "Correctional Health Care in the Texas Department of Criminal Justice." Government West. www.govwest.com (May/June 2001; May 17, 2003).

Ramo, Joshua Cooper. "Doc in a Box." *Time* (Fall 1996): 55–57.

Rapapport, Lisa. "Long-Distance Docs." sacbee.com (February 28, 2003; March 18, 2003).

Research, Training, and Practical Applications: A Look at Developing Programs at the University of Texas Medical Branch at Galveston: Interview with Vincent E. Friedewald. Telehealth.net (2003; May 17, 2003).

Ricci, M. A. "The Vermont Tele-trauma Project: Initial Results" (Abstract). tie.telemed.org (April 2003; May 24, 2003)

Rohland, Barbara. "The Impact of Telemedicine on the Delivery of Psychiatric Services to Rural Areas." Telemedicine Projects: Psychiatric Services. http://telemed/medicine. uiowa.edu/TRCDocs/Projects/impact.html, pp. 1–2 (1998; October 9, 2003).

Salamone, Salvatore. "VPN Eases Meetings of the Mind." *PC World,* June 15, 1998, pp. 1, 78.

Savkar, Sonya, and Robert J. Waters. "Telemedicine—Implications for Patient Confidentiality and Privacy." *Arent Fox Telemedicine Newsletter,* Issue 1. http://www.arentfox.com/telemed/articles/licenseimplic.html#article2, pp. 4–7 (1995; June 8, 1999).

Schwamm, Lee. "Treating Stroke at a Distance Using Telemedicine Could Save Lives, Money." ABCNews.com (February 21, 2003; May 14, 2003).

"Secretary Shalala Announces National Telemedicine Initiative," U.S. National Library of Medicine NIH News Alert, October 8, 1996. http://www.nlm.nih.gov/news/ press_releases/telemed.html, pp. 1–9 (1996; October 9, 2003).

Shepard, Scott. "Telemedicine Brings Memphis Healing to Third-World Patients." Memphis.bizjournals.com (January 17, 2003; May 28, 2003).

Telehealth Update: Final HIPAA Privacy Rules, Office of Advanced Technology. telehealth.hrsa.gov/pubs/hipaa.htm (February 20, 2001; May 15, 2003).

Telemedicine Programs Database. tie.telemed.org (2003; April 8, 2003).

"Telemedicine Report to Congress." January 31, 1997. http://www.ntia.doc.gov/reports/telemed/intro.htm, pp. 1–5 (January 31, 1997; October 9, 2003).

"'Teleoncology' Benefits Cancer Patient in Rural Manitoba; Video-Conferencing Facilitates Consultations between Clinicians and Patients without Travel." cancercare.mb.ca (February 27, 2003; May 28, 2003).

Tufts University Department of Medicine, Massachusetts Telehealth Access Program. www.ntia.doc.gov/otiahome/top/research/exemplary/tufts.htm (2001; May 17, 2003).

Turisco, Fran, Tania Shahid, and L. Paoli. "Technology Use in Rural Health Care: California Survey Results." tie.telemed.org (April 2003; May 25, 2003).

Turner, Janine. "Telepsychiatry as a Case Study of Presence: Do You Know What You Are Missing?" *JCMC* 6 no. 4 (2001). http://www.ascusc.org/jcmc/vol6/issue4/turner.html (July 2001; October 15, 2003).

2001 Report to Congress on Telemedicine, Telehealth. hrsa.gov/pubs/report2001 (May 16, 2002; October 9, 2003).

Tye, Larry. "A High-Tech Link to Boston Aids Vineyard Stroke Victims." neuro-oas.mgh.harvard.edu/stopstroke/Globe_July2001.htm (July 10, 2001; May 14, 2003).

VA Technology Assessment Program Short Report Physiologic Telemonitoring in CHF. med.va.gov (January 2001; June 16, 2003).

Wachter, Glenn. "Telemedicine Legislative Issue Summary: Interstate Licensure for Telenursing." tie.telemed.org (May 2002; March 8, 2003).

RELATED WEB SITES

The American Telemedicine Association (http://www.atmeda.org) is a nonprofit association "promoting greater access to medical care via telecommunications technology." It provides almost unlimited information on the latest developments in telemedicine.

Arent Fox (http://www.arentfox.com) is an excellent source of information on legislative matters relating to telemedicine.

The Center for Telemedicine Law (http://www.ctl.org), a nonprofit organization, "distributes information and serves as a resource on legal issues related to telemedicine."

The National Library of Medicine (http://www.nlm.nih.gov) can provide you with access to a great deal of information including bibliographies.

Telemedicine and Telehealth Networks: The Newsmagazine of Distance Healthcare (http://www.telemedmag.com) is a journal covering the field. Online access to past issues is free.

The University of Iowa's Telemedicine Resource Center (http://telemed.medadmin.uiowa.edu/TRCDocs/trc.html) coordinates the National Laboratory for the Study of Rural Telemedicine.

CHAPTER 5

Information Technology in Radiology

OUTLINE

- **Learning Objectives**
- **Introduction**
- **X-rays**
- **Ultrasound**
- **Digital Imaging Techniques**
  - *Computerized Tomography*
  - *Magnetic Resonance Imaging*
  - *Positron Emission Tomography*
  - *Bone Density Tests*
- **Bloodless Surgery**
- **Selected Reading**
- **Chapter Summary**
- **Key Terms**
- **Review Questions**
  - *Multiple Choice*
  - *True/False Questions*
  - *Critical Thinking*
- **Sources**

LEARNING OBJECTIVES

Upon completion of this chapter, you will be able to

- Describe the contributions of digital technology to imaging techniques.
- List the uses of traditional X-rays and the advantages of digital X-rays.
- Discuss the definition and uses of ultrasound.
- Discuss the newer digital imaging techniques of CT scans, MRIs, Functional MRIs, and PET scans, their uses, and advantages and disadvantages.
- Describe new interventional radiology techniques of bloodless surgery.

INTRODUCTION

The purpose of this chapter is to give students in the health care fields an idea of the extent and impact of information technology in the field of radiology—the branch of medicine that uses X-rays to diagnose and treat disease. This chapter focuses on digital imaging techniques.

The new imaging techniques use computers to generate pictures of internal organs of the body. A digital image is an image in a form computers can process and store in binary digits. Computers can make pictures out of mathematical information. The technical methods used by computers to generate the mathematical information are very complex and beyond the scope of this text. This introduction presents a short survey of the older imaging techniques like **X-ray** and **ultrasound** and the newer technologies that use computer technology, including **computerized tomography** (**CT** scan), **magnetic resonance imaging (MRI)**, and **positron emission tomography** (**PET** scan).

Although the focus of the chapter is on digital imaging techniques, radiology is also concerned with treatment. Interventional radiologists treat disease without surgery. They are now able to open blocked blood vessels and do other procedures. The line between radiology and surgery is changing as **bloodless surgery** and **gamma knife surgery** (which does not involve cutting) become more and more widely used. As images become more and more accurate and complete, as they have during the past twenty years, the field of radiology has become increasingly involved with treatment as well as diagnosis. Interventional radiologists currently treat aneurysms and artherosclerosis, and perform bloodless surgeries on tumors. These issues are touched on briefly below.

Precise, detailed images and image-guided therapies are slowly replacing invasive procedures such as cystoscopies and—in the near future—colonoscopies. Radiological screening for diseases has decreased the need for exploratory surgeries, leading to more timely diagnosis and treatment. Research continues into more and more sophisticated imaging techniques, which promise to change some aspects of clinical medicine (*JAMA*, 2001).

X-RAYS

Digital technology is radically transforming the field of radiology. Not only are new imaging techniques (CT scans, MRIs, PET scans) available, but also older procedures such as X-rays and ultrasound are making use of the new technology. A traditional X-ray uses high-energy electromagnetic waves to produce a two-dimensional picture on film. If the X-ray encounters bone, which it cannot penetrate, this appears white on the film. Whatever organ the X-ray passes through appears black on the film. Some soft tissue appears gray. Contrast agents can improve the clarity of the images, but X-rays do not produce good images of all organs and cannot see behind bones at all.

Digital images have several advantages over images on film. Digital X-rays do not have to be developed, but are immediately available and can be viewed directly on a computer screen, making them accessible to more than one person at a time, that is, to anyone on a computer network. They are more flexible. Areas can be enhanced, emphasized and highlighted, and made larger or smaller. The quality of a copy of a digital X-ray is as good as the quality of the original. Digital X-rays can be immediately transmitted over phone lines for a second opinion. In the future, it is hoped that by taking more than one picture, the X-ray image can be three dimensional.

X-rays still dominate in several areas. If a broken bone is suspected, an X-ray is likely. Most dentists still depend on traditional X-rays, although digital imaging is becoming more widely used. Digital X-rays use less radiation than conventional X-rays. For a digital X-ray, a highly sensitive sensor containing a microchip is put into the patient's mouth. Because it is so sensitive, less radiation can be used. The data is sent to the computer, which displays an image on the monitor within a few seconds. The image can be manipulated, highlighted, enlarged, and shared on a network. The quality of the image is no better than a traditional X-ray, but it does expose patients to less radiation. However, the equipment that is required is still quite expensive.

At the present time, a major imaging area dominated by traditional X-rays is mammography, although this may be changing. In 2000, the FDA approved the first digital mammography system. Ultrasound, which can distinguish between harmless cysts and tumors, may be used with mammograms. Other digital imaging techniques may also be used if an abnormality is spotted by a mammogram. But even with the traditional X-ray, computers can play a part. Computer software has been developed that can be used to reexamine mammogram films, perhaps decreasing the percentage of women whose mammograms are read by radiologists as cancer-free, but who do in fact have malignant tumors. An FDA-approved scanner can further evaluate breast abnormalities found by a mammogram. It is connected to a computer, which displays an image of the breast based on differences in the flow of electricity in normal versus malignant tissue.

ULTRASOUND

Ultrasound technology predates computers by many years. However, it now makes use of computers to create dynamic images. Unlike X-rays, ultrasound uses no radiation. It uses very high frequency sound waves and the echoes they produce when they hit an object. This information is used by a computer to generate an image, producing a two-dimensional moving picture on a screen. Ultrasound is most closely identified with examining a moving fetus. It is also used to study blood flow and to diagnose gallstones and prostate disease. Ultrasound, like other imaging techniques, is being used to decrease the need for surgical biopsies. It has been approved for the treatment of prostate disease.

In 2002, an eleven by six and one-half inch, three-pound handheld ultrasound scanner was developed. The traditional ultrasound is 200–300 pounds. The handheld scanner has a small liquid crystal display. It is easy to use in a doctor's office or emergency room and can be taken to battlefields and accident scenes (Marriott, 2002).

DIGITAL IMAGING TECHNIQUES

Sophisticated imaging machinery uses computers to reduce massive amounts of mathematical data, generated in various ways, to pictures. The pictures that the computer constructs are clearer than traditional X-rays. In addition, the increased use of digital technology has produced the kinds of images that were not possible with traditional X-rays, including three-dimensional representations; pictures that clearly distinguish soft tissue within the body; images of function, change, and movement; and images of the electrical and chemical processes in the brain.

The machinery needed to produce CT scans, MRIs, and PET scans is very expensive compared with the equipment needed for X-rays and ultrasound. However, by providing a clearer, more detailed, and accurate picture of the inside of the body, sophisticated diagnostic imaging is reducing the need for exploratory surgery and reducing cost and hospital stays, along with pain. When surgery is necessary, it may be less traumatic, since it is guided by precise, accurate images. By allowing a view of the activity in the brain, digital imaging techniques are also improving the understanding of the chemical and physical bases of mental illness and aiding in the development of effective medications. Another form of digital imaging is the **SPECT (single photon emission computed tomography)** scan. Like the PET scan, it shows movement. However, SPECT scans are less precise. It is sometimes used because it is less expensive than PET. Because PET and SPECT can be used for similar things, and the SPECT image is not as precise, we have focused on PET scans. Both SPECT and PET scans are classified under nuclear medicine.

Computerized Tomography

Computerized tomography (CT scan) uses X-rays and digital technology to produce a cross-sectional image of the body. CT scans use radiation passing a series of X-rays through the patient's body at different angles. The computer then creates a cross-sectional image from these X-rays. Soft tissue can be distinguished because it absorbs the X-ray differently. A CT scan produces a more useful image than a traditional X-ray. In addition, CT scans can be used to locate nerve centers, thus helping in the reduction of pain. In enhanced CT scans, a dye is used. Enhanced CT scans are used to show brain tumors: Compounds cannot cross normal blood vessels in the brain; abnormal vessels let substances through, including the dye. This can be seen on a CT scan. CT scans help diagnose other conditions, including severe acute respiratory syndrome (SARS). In 2003, a virtual cystoscopy using CT scans was developed to screen for bladder tumors. A traditional cystoscopy is invasive and involves inserting a probe into the bladder, but this does not allow a complete examination. In a virtual cystoscopy, a CT scan of the bladder, an expert uses an image-processing algorithm for help in locating tumors (Sylvain et al., 2003). CT scans are also being used to perform virtual colonoscopies; however, the results still need to be compared with the results of real colonoscopies.

A variation of the traditional CT scan, called the **Ultrafast CT** scan, may be used in place of coronary angiograms to examine coronary artery blockages. Compared with a coronary angiogram, the Ultrafast CT is painless, less dangerous, noninvasive, and less expensive.

Magnetic Resonance Imaging

Magnetic resonance imaging (MRI) machines use computer technology to produce images of soft tissue within the body that could not be pictured by traditional X-rays. Unlike CT scans, MRIs can produce images of the insides of bones. Using a technique called **scientific visualization**, MRI machines use computers and a very strong magnetic field and radio waves to produce pictures. The images are constructed from mathematical data generated by the interaction of radio waves and the protons inside the nuclei of hydrogen atoms in the water and fatty tissue in the human body. The MRI machine creates a magnetic field many times stronger than the earth's; it then generates radio waves. The response of the body's cells is measured by a computer, which uses this data to create an image. Magnetic resonance imaging can produce accurate and detailed pictures of the structures of the body and the brain, and can distinguish between normal and abnormal tissue. MRI is more accurate than other imaging methods for detecting cancer that has spread to the bone. Although PET/CT finds cancer of the lungs more accurately, MRIs may be used for diagnosis and for the treatment of certain conditions that used to require surgery. For example, using MRI, radiologists can now clean or close off arteries without surgery. MRIs do not use radiation and are noninvasive. MRIs are used to image brain tumors and in helping to diagnose disorders of the nervous system such as multiple sclerosis (MS). MRIs also detect stroke at an earlier stage than other tests. MRIs can help find brain abnormalities in patients suffering from dementia (MRI of the Head, 2003). It is particularly useful with brain disorders because it can distinguish among different types of nerve tissue. In 2003, MRIs were used to study comatose patients, and were able to detect normal brain activity (Zimmer, 2003). A new technique will attempt to use MRIs in combination with lasers for instant bloodless high-resolution biopsies. High-powered, pulsed lasers are focused on cells. This gives the cells the ability to glow. Computer software is then used to create a picture of the location of the beam and fluorescence of the cells. Any change in the cell is seen. Because this technique cannot see far into the body, MRIs must be used for a complete picture. Scientists hope to develop an endoscope that can be used for any part of the body.

Relatively new, **functional MRIs** measure small changes in the use of oxygen in an active part of the brain. FMRIs identify brain activity by changes in blood oxygen. The fMRI can be used to identify brain area by function in the operating room and help the surgeon avoid damaging areas such as those that are associated with speech. Strokes, brain tumors, or injuries can change the areas of the brain where functions such as speech, sensation, and memory occur. FMRIs can help locate these areas and can then be used to help develop treatment plans. They can also help in the treatment of brain tumors and the assessment of the effects of stroke, injury, or other disease on brain function. FMRIs are currently being used to study conditioned response in people—what the brain does when learning to associate a stimulus, such as a bell or an image, with food. They are also being used along with PET scans to study schizophrenia (Functional MR Imaging, 2003).

A new experimental technique modifies the conventional MRI. It is called dynamic contrast-enhanced MRI. This technology is being studied in research institutions. It can take 1,000 images of a tumor before, during, and after dye is introduced. Software analyzes the images. It can reveal new tiny blood vessels and how permeable they are. (Blood vessels that feed tumors are full of holes.) If this technique can be perfected, it will be able to show the growth of new blood vessels that feed cancerous tumors at an early stage, and thus give scientists more information to help develop drugs to inhibit the growth of blood vessels (Eisenberg, 2003).

Positron Emission Tomography

Positron emission tomography (PET) scans use radioisotope technology to create a picture of the body in action. PET scans use computers to construct images from the emission of positive electrons (positrons) by radioactive substances administered to the patient. PET scans—unlike traditional X-rays and CT scans—produce images of how the body works, not just how it looks. PET scans may help detect changes in cell function (disease) before changes in structure can be seen by other imaging techniques (Mount Sinai, 2003). PET scans create representations of the functioning of the body and the mind. They are used to study Alzheimer's, Parkinson's, epilepsy, learning disabilities, moral reasoning, bipolar disorder, and cancer. PET scans are also used to diagnose arterial obstructions. They are accurate and can avoid invasive catheterization (Mount Sinai, 2003).

Full body PET scans have been shown effective in detecting the spread of breast cancer. Without the scan 36 percent of tumors were thought to have spread; the scans showed that 52 percent had spread. In general, PET scans have proved superior in diagnosing and staging cancer. They are also used to look for recurrence and for recommending changes in treatment. A combination of CT and PET scans are most effective in detecting cancerous tumors of the lung and lymph nodes—tumors that MRIs missed (Susman, 2002).

A recent study has found that PET scans can measure an esophageal cancer patient's response to chemotherapy and radiation therapy before surgery. PET scans can detect metastases that other imaging techniques could not see. They might in the future be able to predict survival rates ("PET Scans Detect Therapy Responses in Esophagial Cancer Patients," 2003).

Additionally, PET scans can show the functioning of the brain by measuring cerebral blood flow. PET scans produce a picture of activity, of function. A person is administered a small amount of radioactive glucose. The active area of the brain uses the glucose more quickly, and this is reflected in the image that the computer constructs. Neuroimaging techniques using PET can present a picture of brain activity associated with cognitive processes such as memory and the use of language. PET scans are used to study the chemical and physiological processes that take place in the brain when a person speaks correctly or stutters. PET scans can show the specific brain activity associated with schizophrenia, manic-depression, posttraumatic stress disorder, and obsessive-compulsive disorder. They have shown the precise area of the brain that malfunctions in certain mental illnesses and the effects of both drugs such as Prozac and traditional talking therapy on nerve cells. With PET, a picture of a drug's effect on brain function can be developed. They can now predict which patient will be helped by which medication. Because these pictures are anatomically and physiologically exact, they should help in the development of new psychiatric drugs.

In a study in 2002, Dr. Lewis Baker compared the effects of psychotropic medications and talk therapy on patients with obsessive-compulsive disorder. Using PET scans of the brain, he found that the two very different treatments produce similar effects on brain function (Friedman, 2002).

PET scans have even been used to shed light on an issue that philosophers have been concerned with for centuries: moral reasoning. In 2002, a study examined the areas of the brain involved in solving moral dilemmas. When a group of people were asked if they would throw a switch that would kill one person to save five others, most said yes. But when asked if they would personally push one person to his death to save five others, most said no. PET scans showed that depending on how the question was phrased different areas of the brain were brought into action. The first question was stated impersonally, and the reasoning part of the brain was engaged. The second question was asked personally and the emotional part of the brain was engaged (Blakeslee, 2001).

Software packages help researchers study the effects of drugs by combining PET and MRI, allowing them to correlate the functional information from PET-scan images of brain activity with the anatomical details acquired by MRI scans. Studies of the effects of certain drugs (including alcohol and cocaine) on the brain may make use of the precise image of brain structure that magnetic resonance imaging produces and the picture of the functioning of the brain that PET can give us.

Brain imaging techniques, including both PET scans and FMRIs, are aiding in the comprehension of schizophrenia. People with schizophrenia are tormented by auditory hallucinations; their suffering is so great that sometimes it results in suicide. Some psychiatrists have ignored the voices and the content of the messages. However, in 2003, scientists began using FMRIs to correlate the hallucinations to the activity of specific areas of the brain. They found increased activity in areas involved in hearing, speech, emotion, and memory. This has led to a discussion of new theories about schizophrenia. One new treatment has been developed. The treatment involves sending low-frequency magnetic pulses to areas of the brain identified by MRIs as active during hallucinations. It gives temporary relief to patients who don't respond to standard medications (Goode, "Experts See Mind's Voices . . . ," 2003).

The newly approved Given® Diagnostic Imaging System does not fit into any of our categories. It is a capsule with a video camera, lights, transmitter, and batteries. The patient swallows the capsule, which takes pictures of the small intestine, sending them to a small recorder on the patient's belt. After eight to 72 hours the capsule passes out of the digestive track, and the health care provider analyzes the pictures. This device cannot be used on anyone wearing an implantable medical device like a pacemaker.

Bone Density Tests

Osteoporosis is a condition of weak bones. Bones lose mineral content or density. Osteoporosis increases the risk of hip and spine fractures. Some bone loss is a normal accompaniment of aging. Several kinds of tests can be done to diagnose this condition. A bone density scan or dual X-ray absorptiometry (DEXA) scan is a special kind of low radiation X-ray that shows changes in the rays' intensity after passing through bone. Doctors can see small changes in bone density from the amount of change in the X-ray. Quantitative computed tomography creates a three-dimensional image of a skeleton. CT scans are used to measure the amount by which beams of radiation lose power (attenuate) as they pass through matter. This measures the mineral content of bones. Quantitative ultrasound is used, but it is not as accurate a test.

BLOODLESS SURGERY

The effects of digital technology on the practice of medicine cannot be overestimated. As images become more precise, they can guide surgeons better and thus operations are less invasive. In addition, conditions that once required surgery may be amenable to treatment by **interventional radiology**. Some biopsies can now be done with a needle instead of surgically. Stereotactic breast biopsies make use of digital X-rays to locate the abnormality and use a needle to extract tissue. They are less invasive than surgical biopsies, but not as accurate and cannot be used with all patients.

Among the developments in radiology is radiosurgery. On the borderline between radiology and surgery, **stereotactic radiosurgery** (**gamma knife surgery**) is a noninvasive technique that is currently used to treat brain tumors in a one-day session. The use of the gamma knife for brain surgery has grown exponentially over the last few years. It is appropriate for brain tumors because the head can be completely immobilized. It may be used to treat other parts of the body in a different form called fractionated stereotactic radiosurgery; this is delivered over weeks of treatment (Stereotactic Radiosurgery, 2003). Radiosurgery can be performed by a modified linear accelerator that rotates around the patient's head and delivers blasts of radiation to the tumor or by a gamma knife. Called a painless, bloodless surgical device, the gamma knife works by delivering 201 focused beams of radiation directly at the tumor. This kills the tumor and spares the surrounding tissue. The procedure makes use of three-dimensional imaging that locates the tumor in the body and uses computerized targeting to make sure that the center of the tumor gets the most radiation. One published review of the cases of 55 patients found radiosurgery to be quite effective. The newest interventional radiography equipment allows nonsurgical repair of some thoracic abnormalities. The gamma knife is appropriate for some benign brain tumors and all malignant brain tumors. It is also being used to treat neuralgia, intractable pain, Parkinson's, and epilepsy. Some of the advantages of gamma knife surgery involve its relatively low cost, the lack of pain to the patient, the elimination of the risks of hemorrhage and infection, and the short hospital stay. Patients are able to resume daily activities immediately. However, as the procedure grows in popularity, some doctors are questioning its safety and efficacy.

What will the effects of high doses of radiation be in the long run? Although it is recognized as effective in treating some brain tumors, its widespread use is questioned (Okun et al., 2001; Tarkan, 2003).

Research is being done on the effects of ultrasound on malignancies. **Focused ultrasound surgery** does not involve cutting, but rather the use of sound waves. Studies involve the use of ultrasound to stop massive bleeding and to treat cancer. By focusing an ultrasonic beam roughly 10,000 times the power used for prenatal pictures, the temperature of cancerous tissue at the focal point can be raised to nearly boiling. Within seconds, the tissue dies. The main disadvantage is that it cannot be focused through bone (Emerging Technologies Meeting, 2002).

SELECTED READING

Erica Goode. "Brain Imaging May Detect Schizophrenia in Early Stages." *New York Times,* December 11, 2002.

IN THE NEWS

Brain Imaging May Detect Schizophrenia in Early Stages

by Erica Goode

Scientists have known for some time that people who suffer from schizophrenia show abnormalities in the structure of their brains.

But in a new study, researchers for the first time have detected similar abnormalities in brain scans of people who were considered at high risk for schizophrenia or other psychotic illnesses but who did not yet have full-blown symptoms. Those abnormalities, the study found, became even more marked once the illness was diagnosed.

The subjects in the study who went on to develop psychoses had less gray matter in brain areas involved in attention and higher mental processes like planning, emotion and memory, the researchers found.

Experts said the study's results, reported yesterday in an online version of *The Lancet,* the medical journal, offered the possibility that imaging techniques might eventually be used to predict who will develop schizophrenia, a devastating illness that affects more than 2.8 million Americans. Doctors could then offer treatment while the disease was still in its earliest stages, possibly preventing further damage to the brain.

But Dr. Christos Pantelis, an associate professor of psychiatry at the University of Melbourne and the lead author of the report, cautioned that much more research was needed before magnetic resonance imaging, the method used in the study, could serve as a diagnostic tool for individual people with schizophrenia.

(continued)

Brain Imaging May Detect Schizophrenia in Early Stages (*continued*)

"I think it's still too early to say how helpful it will be," Dr. Pantelis said.

Still, other researchers called the study's findings exciting and said that the areas of the brain in which the abnormalities were found would now be an active focus for study.

"This is a terrific first step," said Dr. Paul Thompson, a professor of neurology at the University of California at Los Angeles and an expert on brain imaging and schizophrenia.

Dr. Herbert Y. Meltzer, a professor of psychiatry at Vanderbilt University and an expert on schizophrenia, said, "It proves that the psychosis is almost a late stage in the evolution of the disease process."

He added, "The key message is that this is a neurodevelopmental disorder and that changes in memory, learning, attention and executive decision-making precede the experience of the psychosis."

People who suffer from schizophrenia typically experience auditory hallucinations and have blunted emotional responses and difficulty with activities that require planning or other higher-level processes.

Some studies have suggested that the earlier the illness is treated with antipsychotic drugs the better the prognosis. At least two research groups, one led by Dr. Patrick McGorry, an author of the *Lancet* report, and another at Yale, are conducting studies in which young people who are experiencing some symptoms but have not yet developed schizophrenia are treated with antipsychotic drugs. But the studies have been controversial because it is not yet clear which symptoms predict later illness.

In the new study, the researchers used magnetic resonance imaging to scan the brains of 75 people who were deemed "at high risk" for psychosis because they had a strong family history of severe mental illness or had other risk factors, including transient or mild symptoms of mental disturbance or a decline in mental functioning.

Over the next 12 months, 23 of the subjects developed a full-blown psychosis and 52 did not fall ill, the researchers found.

A comparison of the brain scans from the two groups revealed significant differences in the volume of gray matter in areas of the frontal and temporal lobes and the cingulate gyrus. All three regions have been linked to schizophrenia by previous research, Dr. Pantelis said.

When the researchers conducted additional brain scans on some subjects who developed psychoses, they found further reductions in gray matter not seen in the scans taken before the illnesses were diagnosed.

CHAPTER SUMMARY

- During the past 20 years, imaging techniques have become more precise and accurate due to computer technology. X-rays that image bones and ultrasound, which shows moving images, have been supplemented by computer-based techniques.
- The CT scan takes many images and combines them in a two- or three-dimensional slice.
- The MRI uses magnetism to image soft tissue. Functional MRIs can see small metabolic changes in the brain and can be used to map brain function.
- The PET scan images function. PET can allow the radiologist to see the difference between normal and cancerous cells, and can be used to study brain function in normal and mentally ill patients. PET can watch the brain think and judge.
- The use of these detailed and accurate images has made diagnosis more accurate and exploratory surgery rare.
- Radiology has moved from diagnosis to treatment, using radiosurgery to treat brain tumors and focused ultrasound to treat other kinds of tumors.

KEY TERMS

bloodless surgery
computerized
    tomography (CT)
focused ultrasound
    surgery
functional magnetic
    resonance imaging
    (FMRI)

gamma knife surgery
interventional radiology
magnetic resonance
    imaging (MRI)
positron emission
    tomography (PET)
scientific visualization

SPECT (single photon
    emission computed
    tomography)
stereotactic radiosurgery
Ultrafast CT
ultrasound
X-ray

REVIEW QUESTIONS

Multiple Choice

1. Which of the following uses sound waves and the echoes they produce when they encounter an object to create an image?
   A. X-rays
   B. Ultrasound
   C. Positron emission tomography
   D. Magnetic resonance imaging

2. _____ study brain function by sensing small changes in oxygen levels.
   A. X-rays
   B. CT scans
   C. Ultrasound
   D. Functional magnetic resonance imaging

3. _____ uses small amounts of radioactive materials to create a picture of the body in action.
    A. X-rays
    B. Ultrasound
    C. Positron Emission Tomography
    D. Magnetic Resonance Imaging

4. _____ takes a series of X-rays at different angles. A computer then creates a cross-sectional image.
    A. X-rays
    B. CT scans
    C. Positron emission tomography
    D. Magnetic resonance imaging

5. _____ can be used to show the functioning of the brain.
    A. X-rays
    B. CT scans
    C. Positron emission tomography
    D. All of the above

6. _____ can image soft tissue and the inside of bones.
    A. X-rays
    B. CT scans
    C. Positron emission tomography
    D. Magnetic resonance imaging

7. An advantage of digital X-rays over traditional film X-rays is _____.
    A. A digital X-ray is available immediately.
    B. A digital X-ray can be enhanced.
    C. Digital X-rays use less radiation.
    D. All of the above

8. _____ creates images from data generated by the interaction of radio waves and the protons in hydrogen atoms in the water in the human body.
    A. X-rays
    B. CT scans
    C. Positron emission tomography
    D. Magnetic resonance imaging

9. If you wanted to study the effect of Prozac on the brain you would use _____.
    A. X-rays
    B. CT scans
    C. Positron Emission Tomography
    D. None of the above

10. _____ is used to picture a moving fetus.
    A. X-rays
    B. Ultrasound
    C. Positron Emission Tomography
    D. Magnetic Resonance Imaging

True/False Questions

1. PET scans can show the different activity in the brain when a person speaks correctly versus when he or she stutters. _____
2. Ultrasound uses radiation to create an image. _____
3. Traditional X-rays image behind bones. _____
4. A disadvantage of PET scans is high cost. _____
5. PET scans are usually used for broken bones. _____
6. Interventional radiology is concerned with the treatment of disease. _____
7. Stereotactic radiosurgery involves removing tumors surgically. _____
8. A gamma knife is used to make incisions _____
9. Dentists still use X-rays, which may be traditional or digital. _____
10. SPECT scans, like PET scans, show the body in motion. _____

Critical Thinking

1. Using MRIs and PET scans, researchers are studying the functioning of the brain. Comment on the possible positive and negative ramifications this could have from developing more effective psychotropic medications to mind control.
2. Advances in radiology are changing the boundary between radiology and surgery so that at times it is difficult to distinguish between the fields. Bloodless surgery (gamma knife surgery) is now used to treat certain brain tumors. What other uses can you imagine?
3. What are the advantages and disadvantages of using digital X-rays in dentistry?
4. When a mammogram is done, it can be read by a technician, checked by special software, and scanned by a computerized scanner. If the image is misread, who is responsible—the technician, the software publisher, and/or the hardware manufacturer?
5. The new digital imaging equipment is becoming more affordable so that more medical institutions can acquire it. Discuss the advantages and disadvantages of each method (CT scans, MRIs, and PET scans).

SOURCES

"ARRS: Computed Tomography Colonography Reduces Radiation Risk in Colon Cancer Screening." *DGNews*. www.pslgroup.com (May 7, 2003; May 20, 2003).

Beardsey, Tim. "Putting Alzheimer's to the Tests." *Scientific American* (February 1995): 12–13.

Blakeslee, Sandra. "Watching How the Brain Works as It Weighs a Moral Dilemma." nyt.com (September 25, 2001; September 25, 2001).

"Bones and Osteoporosis." bones-and-osteoporosis.com (April 1, 2003; June 16, 2003).

"Bone Density Test for Osteoporosis." health.Harvard.edu (2003; June 16, 2003).

Cluett, Jonathan. "What Is a Bone Scan?" http://orthopedics.about.com (n.d.; June 16, 2003).

———. "What Is a DEXA scan (bone density test)?" http://orthopedics.about.com/cs/osteoporosis/a/bonedensitytest.htm#b (n.d.; October 7, 2003).

"Computed Tomography Images Help Radiologists Diagnose SARS." DGNews. www.pslgroup
.com (May 14, 2003; May 20, 2003).

"Computerized Scanner Double-Checks Suspicious Mammograms." www.fda.com (August
1999; June 14, 2003).

Eisenberg, Anne. "What's Next: A Budding Tumor Unmasked by the Vessels That Feed It."
nyt.com (July 24, 2003; October 11, 2003).

———. "What's Next; Lasers Set Cells Aglow for a Biopsy without the Knife." nyt.com
(June 26, 2003; October 11, 2003).

Emerging Technologies Meeting—New Cutting Technologies in Surgery, Institute of Physics
and Engineering in Medicine, International Radiosurgery Support Center. ipem.org
(2002; April 26, 2003).

Encyclopedia of Medical Imaging, Vol. 1. "Attenuation." www.medcyclopaedia.com (n.d.;
June 18, 2003).

———. "Quantitative Computed Tomography." www.medcyclopaedia.com (n.d.; June 18, 2003).

FDA Talk Paper. "FDA Approves First Digital Mammography System." www.fda.gov (January
31, 2000; May 17, 2003).

Foreman, Judy. "Brain Scans Help Doctors Understand Psychiatric Ills." sunspot.net (June
9, 2003; June 9, 2003).

Fox, Peter et al. "A PET study of the neural systems of stuttering." *Nature,* July 11, 1996,
158–62.

"Full Body Scan for Breast Cancer." http://www.abc.net.au (September 7, 2000; June 15, 2003).

Friedman, Richard A. "Like Drugs Talk Therapy Can Change Brain Chemistry." nyt.com
(August 27, 2002; August 31, 2002).

"Functional MR Imaging," radiology info.org (n.d.; April 16, 2003).

Giger, Maryellen, and Charles A. Pelizzari. "Advances in Tumor Imaging." *Scientific American*
(September 1996): 110–12.

Goode, Erica. "Experts See Mind's Voices in New Light." nyt.com (May 6, 2003; May 13, 2003).

———. "Studying Modern-Day Pavlov's Dogs, of the Human Variety." nyt.com (August 26,
2003; September 1, 2003).

Haney, Daniel G. "Brain Study Shows How Cocaine Enslaves." *Star-Ledger,* January 11,
1998, p. 35.

Hooper, Judith. "Targeting the Brain." *Time* (Fall 1996): 46–50.

JAMA. "Opportunities for Medical Research." JAMA.AMA-assn.org (February 7, 2001;
September 25, 2002).

Kevles, Bettyanne. "Body Imaging." *Newsweek* (Winter 1997–1998): 74–76.

Kevles, Bettyanne Holzmann. *Naked to the Bone: Medical Imaging in the Twentieth Century.* New
Brunswick, NJ: Rutgers University Press, 1997.

Khafagi, Frederick A., and S. Patrick Butler. "Nuclear Medicine." *Medical Journal of Australia*
7 (January 2002): 176 1: 27. http://www.mja.com.au (January 2002; October 16, 2003).

Marano, Lou. "Ethics and Mapping the Brain." UPI.com (June 4, 2003; June 9, 2003).

Marriott, Michel. "A Palm-Size Ultrasound Scans Safely in a Flash." nyt.com (October 10,
2002; October 10, 2002).

Motluk, Alison. "Cutting Out Stuttering." *New Scientist,* February 1, 1997, 32–35.

Mount Sinai. "What Is a PET Study of the Heart?" msnyuhealth.org (2003; April 16, 2003).

"MRI of the Head." radiologyinfo.org (2003; April 16, 2003).

New Device Clearance Given® Diagnostic Imaging System—K010312. www.fda.gov (August 1,
2001; June 11, 2003).

Nordenberg, Tamar. "The Picture of Health, It's What's Inside That Counts with X-rays, Other Imaging Methods." *FDA Consumer.* http://www.fda.gov (1999; January 15, 1999).

Okun, M.S., N.P. Stover, T. Subramanian, M. Gearing, B.H. Wainer, C.A. Holder, R.L. Watts, J.L. Juncos, A. Freeman, M.L. Evatt, S.U. Schuele, J.L. Vitek, and M.R. DeLong. "Complications of Gamma Knife Surgery for Parkinson Disease." http://www.ncbi.nlm.nih.gov/entrez/query.fcgi?cmd=Retrieve&db=PubMed&list_uids=11735773&dopt=Abstract (2001; May 13, 2004).

"PET Scans Detect Therapy Responses in Esophagial Cancer Patients." mskcc.org (April 2003; April 16, 2003).

Raichle, Marcus E. "Visualizing the Mind." *Scientific American* (April 1994): 58–64.

Rajendran, Joseph. "Positron Emission Tomography in Head and Neck Cancer" (Abstract). Applied Radiology Online. appliedradiology.com (June 6, 2003; June 15, 2003).

"RSNA MEETING: Safe, Painless, CT Exam May Replace Coronary Angiograms." http://www.pslgroup.com (December 2, 1997; June 15, 2003).

Scott, A.M. "Current Status of Positron Emission Tomography in Oncology" (Abstract). ncbi.nlm.nih.gov (June 2002; June 15, 2003).

Stereotactic Radiosurgery. International Radiosurgery Support Association. www.irsa.org (2002; April 26, 2003).

Susman, Ed. "RSNA: Positron Emission/Computed Tomography Fusion and Magnetic Resonance Imaging Detect Different Cancerous Lesions." *Doctor's Guide.* www.docguide.com (December 9, 2002; June 15, 2003).

Sylvain, Jaume, Matthieu Ferrant, Benoît Macq, Lennox Hoyte, Julia R. Fielding, Andreas Schreyer, Ron Kikinis, and Simon K. Warfield. "Tumor Detection in the Bladder Wall with a Measurement of Abnormal Thickness in CT Scans." *IEEE Transactions on Biomedical Engineering* 50, no. 3 (March 2003): 383–88.

Tarkan, Laurie. "Brain Surgery, without Knife or Blood, Gains Favor." nyt.com (April 29, 2003; April 29, 2003).

Tempany, Clare, and Barbara McNeil. "Advances in Biomedical Imaging." *JAMA* 285 (2001): 562–67.

What's New In—Inside Mount Sinai News. www.mountsinaihospital.org (February 17, 2003; October 7, 2003).

Wu, D. Gambhir. "Positron Emission Tomography in Diagnosis and Management of Invasive Breast Cancer: Current Status and Future Perspectives" (Abstract). PubMed NLM.gov (April 2003; June 15, 2003).

"X-rays Go Digital." *Sun Magazine.* http://www.sun.com.au (August–September 2000; June 15, 2003).

Zimmer, Carl. "What If There Is Something Going on in There?" nyt.com (September 28, 2003; September 29, 2003).

CHAPTER 6

Information Technology in Dentistry

OUTLINE

- **Learning Objectives**
- **Overview**
- **Education**
- **Administrative Applications**
  - *The Electronic Dental Chart*
- **Demographics and the Transformation of Dentistry**
- **Computerized Instruments in Dentistry**
- **Endodontics**
- **Periodontics**
- **Cosmetic Dentistry**
- **Diagnosis and Expert Systems**
- **Diagnostic Tools**
  - *X-rays*
  - *Digital Radiography*
  - *Electrical Conductance*
  - *Emerging Methods*
  - *Light Illumination*
- **Lasers in Dentistry**
- **Minimally Invasive Dentistry**
- **Surgery**
- **The Growth of Specialization**
- **Teledentistry**
- **Selected Reading**
- **Chapter Summary**
- **Review Questions**
  - *Multiple Choice*
  - *True/False Questions*
  - *Critical Thinking*
- **Sources**

LEARNING OBJECTIVES

Upon completion of this chapter, you will be able to

- Describe the use of computers in education.
- Discuss the significance of the electronic patient record in integrating practice management and clinical applications.
- List the impact of changing demographics on dental practice.
- Describe the use of computers in endodontics, periodontics, and cosmetic dentistry.
- Define diagnostic tools, including the X-ray, digital X-ray, electronic concordance, and the new tools that use light.
- Define minimally invasive dentistry.
- List the uses of computers in dental surgery.
- Describe the trend toward growing specialization.
- Describe the emerging field of teledentistry.

OVERVIEW

Computers have been transforming dentistry for many years. **Dental informatics** combines computer technology with dentistry to create a basis for research, education, and the solution of real-world problems in oral health care using computer applications. From the time the patient calls the office for an appointment recorded in an electronic appointment book, to the services offered and the instruments in use, even to the pain the patient senses, digital technology plays a role. The earliest application of information technology in the dentist's office, as in so many other offices, was administrative—related to bookkeeping and accounting.

Today, computer technology can be utilized in dentistry to help train dentists, to facilitate communication between dentists, to manage dental offices, and to enhance patient care.

The practice of dentistry has also been affected by demographic changes in our society over the last century. Younger people (with the significant exceptions of the poor, minorities, and immigrants) have few cavities due to preventive care. Older people are subject to periodontal disease.

EDUCATION

Dentists can surf the Web for online information specific to their professional interests and use e-mail to communicate with each other and their patients. Computer-generated treatment plans are used to help educate patients (Figure 6.1).

Although not yet common, virtual reality simulations are beginning to be used in the education of dentists and dental surgeons. One school that installed virtual dentistry equipment at a cost of $2 million in 2002 is very satisfied with the part virtual reality can play in dental education. The simulators are always available, so students can learn at their own pace. According to faculty members, students learned much faster; they report that students learned drilling techniques in two weeks instead of one full semester. Each station includes a mannequin, drill, syringes, suction, light, cabinets, and a computer monitor—simulating a dentist's office. A camera watches the student's work and sends the student messages. The student is shown what the tooth should look like, and images and evaluations of the student's work via the monitor.

DentSim is a program that uses virtual reality. Its purpose is to teach technical dexterity to dental students. A small pilot study has been completed. The study found that using the program improved technical dexterity. More studies are planned (Urbankova, 2002).

ADMINISTRATIVE APPLICATIONS

From the moment a patient calls to arrange an appointment, to the electronic submission of the bill to the insurance company, computer technology may be involved. Many dental offices, like other medical offices, use computerized appointment calendars; thus appointments can be made (and viewed) from any room in the office that has a networked computer (Figure 6.2). Specialized software helps to create treatment plans, to explain plans to patients, and to give postoperative instructions. In offices using fully integrated practice management software, any screen is accessible from any other, simply by clicking the mouse.

The Electronic Dental Chart

Computers were first used by dentists in the 1960s as accounting tools. In the 1980s, computers were used for practice management. The American Dental Association (ADA) began developing guidelines for the fully integrated computerized dental office. The electronic appointment book, electronic accounting software, and electronic record keeping in which the patient's record includes images, charting, and photos will become more and more common (Figure 6.3). Software that computerizes some clinical procedures (charting, probing, and digital imaging) is beginning to be used. In the future a patient record that links practice management with all clinical procedures may be developed.

The **electronic dental chart** will be standardized, easy to search, and easy to read (Figure 6.4). It will integrate practice management tasks (administrative applications) with clinical information. It will include all of the patient's conditions and treatments, including images. Although no standards currently exist on what should be in a chart, dental charting software is creating a standard record. The record must include codes for treatment and diagnosis; these will come from the ADA. The chart should include the following: the ability to find patients by name, patient identification numbers, health information such as allergies or conditions that would affect dental care, treatment planning, procedures performed and planned, treatments completed, medical history, and ADA codes. As additions are made, they must be dated, and an audit trail of who edited each record must be kept. Files must be password protected. The record includes graphics and text. The chart will be created on a patient's first visit and updated every visit. Not only does it contain clinical

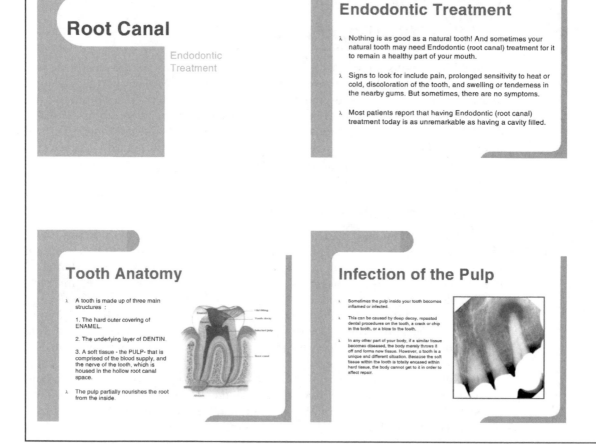

FIGURE 6.1   Software is available to help educate patients about dental treatments. This PowerPoint presentation explains Root Canal Therapy.
Screen shots are from SOFTDENT Practice Management Software. Courtesy of Eastman Kodak Company.

Treatment

It is the role of the dentist to do what the body is unable to do. He must :

- Remove the soft tissue located in the internal spaces (canals).

- Cleanse the area.

- Fill the canals with a special material so that bacteria cannot re-enter the tooth to cause another infection.

Treatment (cont.)

λ The dentist removes the inflamed or infected pulp, carefully cleans and shapes the inside of the tooth, then fills and seals the space.

λ Often it is necessary to place a POST down into the canal space to act as an anchor when large amounts of tooth structure are missing due to disease.

λ While many patients may be in great pain before seeing the dentist, most report that the dentist relieves the pain and that they are comfortable during the procedure.

λ When the endodontic treatment is complete, the tooth is by no means "dead". It receives quite adequate support from the surrounding tissues and may be expected to last as long as any other natural tooth.

Post Op Care

λ For the first few days after treatment, the tooth may feel sensitive - especially if there was pain or infection before the procedure. This discomfort can be relieved with medications.

λ You should not chew or bite on the treated tooth until you have had it restored by your dentist, because it could fracture.

λ Often it is necessary to place a POST down into the canal space to act as an anchor when large amounts of tooth structure are missing due to disease.

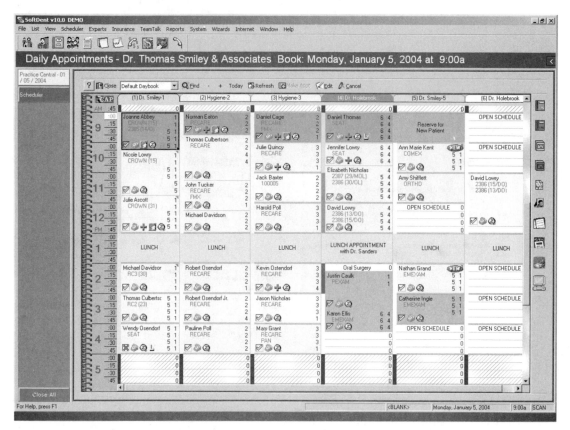

FIGURE 6.2   An appointment can be made in an electronic appointment book.
The screen shot is from SOFTDENT Practice Management Software. Courtesy of Eastman Kodak Company.

information, but also transactions can be posted. It includes the fee schedule and patient's insurance information (including copayment and deductible). Because much of the chart is images, it is easy for the patient to understand. The patient and dentist can develop treatment plans that take into account medical needs and finances. The chart can be electronically transmitted to specialists.

DEMOGRAPHICS AND THE TRANSFORMATION OF DENTISTRY

In the year 2000, the surgeon general issued a first report on dental health. The report pointed to changes over the last 100 years. In the year 1900, most people lost their teeth by middle age. By the middle of the twentieth century, the baby boom generation was taught to take care of their teeth. Bacteria (usually streptococcus) were found to be the cause of tooth decay and periodontal disease in the 1950s and 1960s.

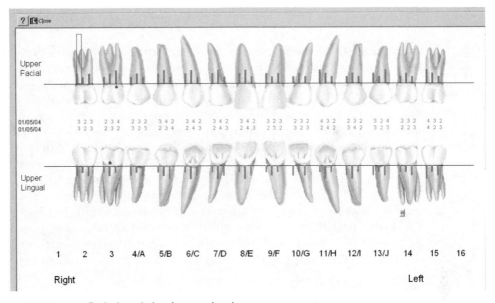

FIGURE 6.3 Periodontal charting can be done on a computer screen.
The screen shot is from SOFTDENT Practice Management Software. Courtesy of Eastman Kodak Company.

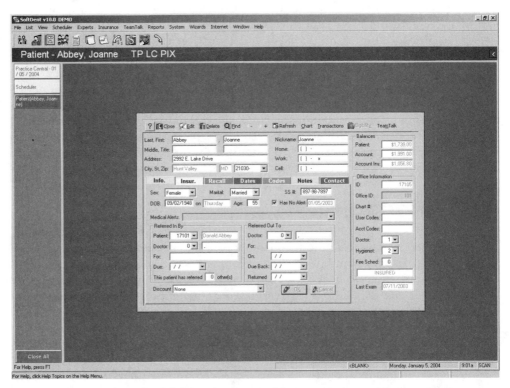

FIGURE 6.4 All of a patient's information is accessible on any computer on the network.
The screen shot is from SOFTDENT Practice Management Software. Courtesy of Eastman Kodak Company.

By the late twentieth century, many children were drinking fluoridated water, having their teeth regularly cared for, and thus suffering less decay. This meant that they did not lose their teeth as they aged. However, according to the surgeon general, there is still an "epidemic of oral disease." Victims of this epidemic are low-income, minority, and some immigrant populations. One study traced the high number of cavities in poor children to increased lead levels in the children's blood, plus shortages in calcium and vitamin C (Carpenter, 1999). But dental health in general has improved over the last century. These trends—successful preventive treatments.in middle-class children and an increasing aging population who have kept their teeth—have changed the conditions dentists are treating and the expectations of patients. Dentists are filling fewer teeth, but increasingly and aggressively treating the more affluent portion of the aging population. This population now seeks dental care to save their teeth. However, this may make the dentist's job more difficult because this population is both old and may be in poor health.

COMPUTERIZED INSTRUMENTS IN DENTISTRY

Computerized instruments have been entering the field of dentistry for several years. From a very expensive machine that creates crowns immediately to fiber-optic digital cameras and digital X-rays, computer technology is changing some aspects of dentistry. The **fiber-optic camera** is analogous to the endoscope used in surgery. See Chapter 7 for a complete discussion of the use of endoscopes in surgery. It is used to view an area that is normally difficult to see. The dentist aims a fiber-optic wand at the area of the mouth to be examined. The image can be viewed on a monitor by patient and dentist. The image can help the dentist see and diagnose problems at a very early stage. An electronic periodontal probe has been developed to replace the sharp steel probe dentists use to measure pockets between teeth. It is more accurate and, one would hope, less painful than its predecessor.

ENDODONTICS

According to the American Dental Association, **endodontics** is the dental specialty that diagnoses and treats diseases of the pulp. Endoscopes make use of fiber optics to take pictures of the root canal and show them on a screen. Both dentist and patient can see and discuss the images. This helps in both diagnosis and educating the patient.

The precision of ultrasonic instruments helps in performing root canal therapy. They are flexible and accurate, and allow the dentist to clean out the root without harming surrounding tissue.

If a patient needs a crown, computers can be used to create a model of the affected tooth. This computer-generated model can be electronically transmitted to another company that uses it to prepare the crown. Too expensive to be common, CAD/CAM is used by a new machine to create crowns.

PERIODONTICS

According to the American Dental Association, **periodontics** is concerned with diagnosing and treating diseases of the gums and other structures supporting the teeth. Periodontal disease is more prevalent in older people who have kept their natural teeth. The standard method of measuring periodontal pockets (the spaces between teeth and gums) involves probing with a steel-tipped tool, measuring the pockets, and noting the depth on a patient's chart. An electronic probe with a flexible tip may be more accurate and less painful.

The change in the conditions for which people seek dental care is related to the demographic changes mentioned earlier. Older adults with their own teeth are more likely to suffer from periodontal disease. Gums recede; roots are exposed and may develop cavities. The more teeth a person keeps, the more these problems develop, the more visits to the dentist. Further, affluent older adults may seek cosmetic dentistry: "smile makeovers," tooth whitening, and orthodontics.

COSMETIC DENTISTRY

Cosmetic dentistry attempts to create a more attractive smile. To do this, several procedures may be employed. Tooth bleaching may be done at home with bleaching kits or at the dentist's office using lasers. Porcelain veneers may be applied to create a whiter looking tooth. **Bonding** involves the application of a material to the tooth that can be shaped and polished. **Dental implants** can be used to replace missing teeth; computers help plan the exact placement of the implant. Cosmetic dentists and orthodontists employ digital cameras and graphics software. This allows the patient to view her or himself before and after any procedure. Some software even morphs the image—from the face before to the face after—to show the patient how his or her face will be changed by the procedure. The dental hygienist photographs the patient using a digital camera, and simply makes the changes by dragging the mouse on the image of the patient's face on the screen.

DIAGNOSIS AND EXPERT SYSTEMS

Diagnosis is not always clear and simple; dentists need to analyze all sorts of data, such as the clinical presentation of the patient and general medical information. No individual can have all the current information. But knowing how to phrase questions and find facts for decision making is a crucial skill. There are several collections of evidence-based articles and reviews categorized by topic that dentists can search online. Journals such as the *Journal of Evidence-Based Dental Practice* give summaries of articles. Databases such as MEDLINE can also be helpful. When doing the search, the dentist needs to be able to frame questions that provide enough information. The question should state the problem clearly, as well as the desired outcome. The computerized search should be of peer-reviewed, evidence-based relevant material.

The dentist then needs to apply the correct factual information to the particular situation to make a diagnosis. In dentistry as in other fields, expert systems can help. Expert systems are a branch of artificial intelligence, which attempts to model computer logic on human behavior. An expert system maintains a large collection of facts relevant to the discipline (dentistry) and rules on how these facts are used in decision making. The dentist may type in symptoms, and the expert system may respond by asking for more information; finally, diagnoses are suggested. The diagnosis is in the form of an inference: if the patient exhibits swelling, there may be the presence of an infection. Expert systems are meant as an aid in diagnosis, not a replacement for the judgment of the dentist. **EXPERTMD** is software that allows the creation of medical and dental expert systems.

DIAGNOSTIC TOOLS

A basic diagnostic tool is a clinical examination using a probe. This method is not completely accurate. One study found that in 15 percent of teeth that dentists found to be healthy, X-rays found cavities.

X-rays

Traditional X-rays have been used for more than 100 years to diagnose cavities. X-rays are more effective than clinical examination. They can be used because as the mineral content of the tooth decreases, the X-ray shows the cavity as darker. The dentist must then interpret the X-ray correctly. This is not a foolproof method of diagnosis, and may not detect cavities at an early stage when minimal intervention is necessary.

Digital Radiography

As an aid in diagnosis, digital X-rays have some advantages. They take less time and expose the patient to from 60 to 90 percent less radiation (Figures 6.5 and 6.6). There is a cost savings on film and processing. Dentists will no longer have to store film. The image needs no developing and the image can be viewed and enhanced immediately on a monitor by both the dentist and the patient. The patient can see the digital image more clearly than a small film, and aspects of the digital X-ray can be enhanced to show specific problem areas. Computers can be used to scan X-ray images into a patient's digital file. Like the traditional X-ray, the digital X-ray also needs interpretation. Several studies, however, have found no significant differences in diagnosis between digital and traditional imaging.

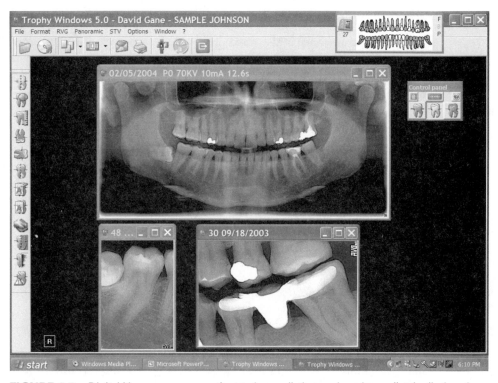

FIGURE 6.5 Digital X-rays expose a patient to less radiation and are immediately displayed on a monitor.
The screen shot is from SOFTDENT Practice Management Software. Courtesy of Eastman Kodak Company.

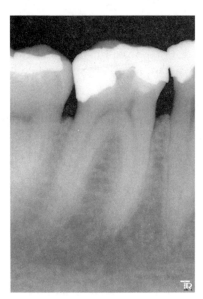

FIGURE 6.6 Digital X-ray.
The screen shot is from SOFTDENT Practice Management Software. Courtesy of Eastman Kodak Company.

Electrical Conductance

Electrical conductance is also currently used to diagnose cavities. An electric current is passed through a tooth, and the tooth's resistance is measured. A decayed tooth has a different resistance reading than a healthy tooth. Studies differ on the accuracy of this method, but tend to rate it high in detecting substantial cavities, not early lesions.

Emerging Methods

Traditional clinical exams and X-rays can detect cavities only after they are somewhat advanced. New methods use light to attempt to identify cavities earlier. Studies disagree on their effectiveness. New techniques have also been developed to stop demineralization, which occurs with caries; however, the success of these treatments is not yet known.

Light Illumination

Several methods use light to help diagnose tooth disease. These show promise in diagnosing early lesions. To find decay, a bright light is used to illuminate the tooth, revealing color differences. Decay looks darker because the light is absorbed when a cavity changes the structure of enamel.

Fiber-optic transillumination found early lesions (affecting enamel), but was limited in diagnosing advanced caries.

Digital Imaging Fiber-Optic Transillumination (DIFOTI®) involves using a digital CCD camera to obtain images of teeth trans-illuminated with white light (Figure 6.7). The images are analyzed using computer algorithms. In NIH-sponsored studies DIFOTI® was more sensitive than radiography for detection of occlusal, interproximal, and smooth surface caries: Occlusal (X-ray 20%, DIFOTI® 80%); Interproximal (X-ray 31%, DIFOTI® 69%); and Smooth surface (X-ray 4%, DIFOTI® 41%) (Schneiderman, A., and M. Elbaum, et al. 1997;31:103–110).

DIFOTI® can find recurrent caries around restorations (amalgams, composites, sealants) and fractures that X-rays could not diagnose. Images are displayed in real-time on a computer monitor for patient education and are stored on a patient database on a PC.

Intra-oral fiber-optic cameras allow both patient and dentist to get a close-up tour of the patient's mouth (Figure 6.8). A fiber-optic device is aimed at an area of the patient's mouth, and the image appears on the screen. The image can be magnified, and thus shows problems, like small cracks, that might otherwise remain unnoticed until the tooth breaks.

LASERS IN DENTISTRY

Laser stands for light amplification by stimulated emission of radiation. Lasers deliver light energy. Depending on the target, the light travels at different wavelengths. Each target absorbs one wavelength and reflects other wavelengths. So each instrument is different. There are several uses of lasers in dentistry. Low-level

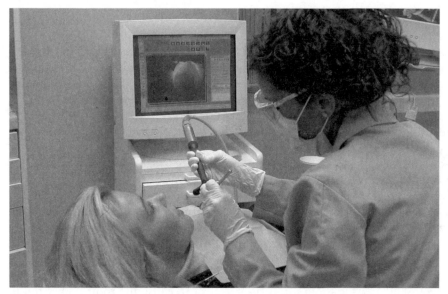

(a)

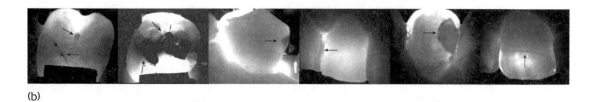

(b)

FIGURE 6.7 (a) Hygienist imaging patient with DIFOTI® system. (b) DIFOTI® images of: 1) virgin occlusal caries, 2) recurrent occlusal caries around amalgam, 3) incipient interproximal decay, 4) incipient interproximal decay, 5) recurrent buccal decay around composite, and 6) horizontal anterior fracture.
Courtesy of DIFOTI®.

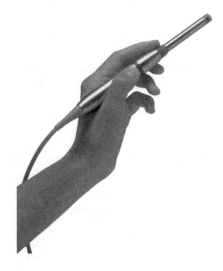

FIGURE 6.8 An intra-oral camera can help reveal problems before they become serious.
Courtesy of Eastman Kodak Company.

lasers can find pits in tooth enamel that may become cavities. The FDA has approved laser machines for drilling and filling cavities; lasers also reduce the bacteria in the cavity. Minimally invasive dentistry uses lasers. Surgical lasers, used in place of drills, burst cells by heating them. One laser works on hard tissue, another on soft tissue. Lasers can quickly harden the material used to fill the tooth, reducing the time a filling takes to complete. Lasers cannot be used where previous fillings or crowns exist.

Lasers are used by periodontists; they can reshape the gums. They can also be used to remove bacteria from periodontal pockets. But their use is limited in root canal therapy. The FDA has approved one laser for treating root canals. Lasers can be used in some instances to help clean out the root canal and to remove bacteria. However, they can only be used in straight canals because the instruments are glass and do not bend. If the temperature is too high, the canal space can be charred, and the tooth and surrounding tissue can be damaged.

Lasers also have uses in cosmetic dentistry. Dentists can apply whitening solutions to teeth and activate them using lasers. This can cause the tooth to lighten in a very short time.

MINIMALLY INVASIVE DENTISTRY

Minimally invasive dentistry emphasizes prevention and the least possible intervention. Teeth are constantly affected by acids, which **demineralize** the surfaces (dissolve the enamel). Early lesions beneath the enamel can be treated with calcium, phosphate, and fluoride, which help **remineralize** teeth (restore the enamel). Preventive measures include antibacterial rinses and toothpastes, fluoride, diet, sealants, and the use of sugarless gum to increase saliva. The widespread use of fluoride has strengthened tooth enamel but not the dentin. Many cavities, which appear in X-rays, are simply not found by traditional clinical examination. Cavities often appear in hard-to-see fissures in a tooth. Sealants may be used as a preventative measure. If a cavity is there, minimally invasive techniques may be used to prepare the tooth. Air abrasion can remove small amounts of a tooth; it involves aiming high-speed particles at the tooth. It can be used for the removal of cavities, of defects in the enamel, and to detect cavities in fissures by opening them for inspection. It is relatively painless. It removes less of the tooth than a traditional drill.

Minimally invasive dentistry also makes use of lasers. Painless lasers can be used in place of the drill to fill cavities. The laser vaporizes decay by directing a stream of light at the affected area. The lasers are so precise that they affect only the decay, not the tooth. Very few patients require pain medication, and those who do are sensitive to the cold water used, not the laser. The machine is much more expensive than the conventional drill, but it allows fillings to be done so quickly that many more patients can be treated.

SURGERY

Computers play a part in dental surgery, from the delivery of anesthesia to the planning and creation of dental implants. Computerized monitoring devices can keep track of a patient's vital signs. For patients requiring implants, software can create a three-dimensional view of the patient. This allows the dentist to see the exact relationship of the planned implant to the patient's bone. The surgery can be done as a simulation; dental CT scans allow the surgeon to rotate the implant on the screen so that by the time the patient is operated on, the surgery is planned down to the last detail. The software can measure bone density from the image and predict whether bone grafts will be needed. Procedures take less time and are easier for both patient and dentist.

THE GROWTH OF SPECIALIZATION

In the last quarter of the twentieth century, only 10 percent of dentists were specialists. This is expected to rise to about 30 percent. This is due in part to the decrease in the number of dentists trained, while the number of specialists trained remains constant, so that specialists form a greater proportion. It is also due to changing demographics. As life expectancy increases and dental health improves, more affluent patients who feel they need to be attractive will seek cosmetic dentistry. With the aging population, some dentists will specialize in geriatrics. New technologies that allow dental problems to be diagnosed and treated earlier will result in dentists who specialize in diagnostics. Group practices may increase. In 2000, 108 million people in the United States lacked dental insurance (Gorman, 2000). However, there is the possibility of the inclusion of dental services under HMOs, which will expect preventive care and economical service. Patients may educate themselves via the Internet and expect more from their dentists.

TELEDENTISTRY

Teledentistry programs have been developed to help dentists access specialists, improving patient care. One system uses the Internet and requires a computer and digital camera. The general dentist can e-mail a patient's chart, including images, to the specialist who can suggest both diagnosis and treatment. This saves the patient time and travel, and gives the patient access to expert advice.

SELECTED READING

Scanlon, Jessie. "Say Ahhh (and Watch the Monitor)." nyt.com (September 4, 2003; September 4, 2003).

IN THE NEWS

Excerpt from "Say Ahhh (and Watch the Monitor)"

by Jessie Scanlon

You sit down, you open your mouth, say ahhh. The dentist leans down and peers in, metal probe in one hand, angled mirror in the other, and starts poking.

[Now] the process [is] a bit different.
. . . [T]he hygienist reviewed [the patient's] chart and images on her flat panel display, then reached for a wandlike device called a Difoti. She positioned it above each tooth. . . . As she did, light passed through the enamel in a process called transillumination. Any cavities or other irregularities altered the light pattern, and the information was captured by the wand's sensor . . . and transmitted to a display that she and [the patient] were watching.

The Difoti . . . is one of a range of new digital technologies . . . [helping to catch] problems sooner. . . .
Lasers, sonar, digital radiography and rapid manufacturing are making dental work more efficient, less painful, and of better quality.

Some dentists . . . say that imaging technologies play an important role in their relationship with patients. . . . [T]he premise is that they will be more willing to go ahead with a root canal if they have witnessed the sorry state of the root.
Another advantage of these powerful detection and imaging techniques is that they can sometimes help to reduce the discomfort of examinations and treatments. . . .
One alternative is the soft-tissue laser. . . . First used for whitening, diode lasers are increasingly being used to shape the gum line and treat gum disease because they are mush kinder to the tissue than a scalpal, and patients require no anesthetic.

September 4, 2003. Copyright © 2003 by The New York Times Company. Reprinted by permission.

CHAPTER SUMMARY

Computers are used in dentistry for the education of both dentists and patients and to assist in dental surgery.

- The electronic patient record may standardize the dental chart and integrate the practice by including all of a patient's information from personal, financial, and insurance to clinical information.

- Changing demographics and improved dental health for most children have combined to change the tasks performed by dentists.
- Computer technology is making the tools used by periodontists, endodontists, and surgeons more precise.
- Cosmetic dentistry attempts to create a more attractive smile using whitening, bonding, and implants.
- Traditional diagnostic tools are being supplemented by methods based on digital technology and fiber optics.
- Minimally invasive dentistry emphasizes prevention and the least possible intervention.
- Computers play a role in dental surgery from delivering anesthesia to monitoring a patient's vital signs.
- Lasers are used in many branches of dentistry including cosmetic dentistry.
- More and more dentists are specializing in a particular field.
- Teledentistry can deliver expert consults at a distance.

KEY TERMS

bonding
cosmetic dentistry
demineralize
dental implants
dental informatics
DentSim
Digital Imaging
    Fiber-Optic
    Transillumination
    (DIFOTI®)

electrical conductance
electronic dental chart
endodontics
EXPERTMD
fiber-optic camera
fiber-optic
    transillumination
intra-oral fiber-optic
    cameras

laser (light amplification
    by stimulated
    emission of
    radiation)
minimally invasive
    dentistry
periodontics
remineralize
teledentistry

REVIEW QUESTIONS

Multiple Choice

1. The _____ is analogous to the endoscope used in surgery.
    A. Digital X-ray
    B. Laser
    C. Fiber-optic camera
    D. None of the above
2. _____ is the dental specialty that diagnoses and treats diseases of the pulp.
    A. Periodontics
    B. Endodontics
    C. Cosmetic dentistry
    D. Digital dentistry

3. _____ is the dental specialty that diagnoses and treats diseases of the gums.
   A. Periodontics
   B. Endodontics
   C. Cosmetic dentistry
   D. Digital dentistry

4. _____ is the dental specialty concerned with smile makeovers.
   A. Periodontics
   B. Endodontics
   C. Cosmetic dentistry
   D. Digital dentistry

5. _____ emphasizes prevention and the least possible intervention.
   A. Periodontics
   B. Endodontics
   C. Cosmetic dentistry
   D. Minimally invasive dentistry

6. _____ can find cavities developing behind metal fillings.
   A. Traditional examination
   B. DIFOTI®
   C. Traditional X-rays
   D. Digital X-rays

7. _____ is software that allows the creation of medical and dental expert systems.
   A. POEMS
   B. MYCIN
   C. INTERNIST
   D. EXPERTMD

8. _____ can remove small amounts of a tooth; it involves high-speed particles aimed at the tooth.
   A. DIFOTI®
   B. Light illumination
   C. Air abrasion
   D. None of the above

9. _____ deliver light energy. Depending on the target, the light travels at different wavelengths.
   A. Lasers
   B. X-rays
   C. Air abrasion
   D. All of the above

10. One study traced the high number of cavities in poor children to _____.
    A. increased lead levels in the children's blood
    B. shortages in calcium
    C. shortages in vitamin C
    D. All of the above

True/False Questions

1. Painless lasers cannot be used in place of the drill to fill cavities. _____
2. Dental health in general has improved over the last century. _____

3. Teeth are constantly affected by acids, which demineralize the surfaces. _____
4. The percentage of dentists who are specialists is not expected to rise. _____
5. The change in the conditions for which people seek dental care is related to demographic changes. _____
6. The laser vaporizes decay by directing a stream of light at the affected area. _____
7. The earliest application of information technology in the dentist's office was administrative—related to bookkeeping and accounting. _____
8. Lasers can always be used in to help clean out the root canal and to remove bacteria. _____
9. Lasers are used in cosmetic dentistry. _____
10. Traditional clinical exams and X-rays can detect cavities only after they are somewhat advanced. _____

Critical Thinking

1. What are the primary functions of computer technology in the dentist's office? In your answer, refer to clinical, administrative, and special purpose applications.
2. How do you envision dentistry 10 years from now?
3. How would you address the need for proper dental care for children who are disadvantaged?
4. What methods would you incorporate to educate people about good oral health care?
5. How would you close the gap between the poor, health care deficient populace and the affluent, who can afford proper, regular dental care?
6. With an aging population, dentistry will have to reflect the demand for cosmetic surgery. Do you think that insurance should cover this? Why or why not?

SOURCES

Alipour-Rocca, L., V. Kudryk, and T. Morris. "A Teledentistry Consultation System and Continuing Dental Education via Internet." *Journal of Medical Internet Research* 1999 (suppl 1): e110. jmir.org (January 1999; March 18, 2003).

American Association of Cosmetic Dentists. "Not Satisfied with Your Smile? You're Not Alone." http://www.aacd.com (July 15, 2002; June 16, 2003).

———. "Seniors Benefit from Cosmetic Dentistry," http://www.aacd.com (June 3, 2002; June 16, 2003).

American Association of Endodontists. "Position Paper on the Use of Lasers in Dentistry." aae.org (April 1, 2000; June 16, 2003).

American Dental Association. "Cosmetic Dentistry." ada.org (1995–2003; June 18, 2003).

Angier, Natalie. "Dentistry, Far Beyond Drilling and Filling." nyt.com (August 5, 2003; August 5, 2003).

Carpenter, S. "Lead and Bad Diet Give a Kick in the Teeth (Poor Children Are Most Susceptible to Lead Toxicity)." *Science News,* findarticle.com (June 26, 1999; June 2, 2003).

Clark, Glenn T. "Teledendistry: Genesis, Actualization, and Caveats." *Journal of the California Dental Association,* CDA Journal. www.cda.org/member/pubs/journal/authors_00.htm (2000; June 3, 2003).

Delrose, Daniel C., and Richard W. Steinberg. "The Clinical Significance of the Digital Patient Record." *JADA* 131 (June 2000): 57s–60s.

"Diagnosis and Management of Dental Caries." Summary, Evidence Report/Technology Assessment: Number 36. AHRQ Publication No. 01-E055. ahrq.gov (February 2001; June 3, 2003).

Douglas, Chester W., and Cherilyn Sheets. "Patients' Expectations of Oral Health in the 21st Century." *JADA* 131 (June 2000): 3s–7s.

Dove, S. Brent. "Radiographic Diagnosis of Dental Caries." uthscsa.edu (n.d.; June 2, 2003).

Drisco, Connie H. "Trends in Surgical and Nonsurgical Periodontal Treatment." *JADA* 131 (June 2000): 31s–38s.

Forrest, J. L., and S. A. Miller. "Evidence-Based Decision Making in Action: Part 1— Finding the Best Clinical Evidence." *J Contemp Dent Pract.* thejcdp.com (August 2002; June 16, 2003).

Freydberg, B. K. "Connecting to Success: Practice Management on the Net." *J Contemp Dent Pract.* thejcdp.com (September 2001; June 16, 2003).

Glickman, Gerald N. "21st-Century Endodontics," *JADA* 131 (June 2000): 39s–46s.

Gorman, Jessica. "The New Cavity Fighters." *Science News.* findarticles.com (August 19, 2000; June 2, 2003).

Goshtasby, Andy. "Construction of Electronic Dental Casts." http://www.cs.wright.edu/people/faculty/agoshtas/nih.html (February 17, 1996; June 12, 2003).

Griffin, Susan. "Virtual Dentistry Becomes Reality in Multimedia Lab." cwru.edu (September 27, 2001; October 13, 2003).

Krusin, Martin. Notes and Conversations with the author. July 2004.

Kurtzweil, Paula. "Dental More Gentle with Painless 'Drillings' and Matching Fillings." *FDA Consumer.* fda.gov (May–June 1999, June 4, 2003).

"Laser Dentistry." floss.com (n.d.; June 16, 2003).

NIH Consensus Statement on Dental Caries Management. ADHA Online. odpod.nih.gov (2003; June 3, 2003).

Palombo, Claudio. "Expert Systems in Dentistry—Editorial." *Online Journal of Dentistry* 2 no. 4. www/epub.org (n.d.; June 16, 2003).

Parks, E. T., and G. F. Williamson. "Digital Radiography: An Overview." *J Contemp Dent Pract.* thejcdp.com (November 2002; June 16, 2003).

Remote Dental Consultation Project. cip.upenn.edu (March 14, 2000; May 16, 2003).

Scanlon, Jessie. "Say Ahhh (and Watch the Monitor)." nyt.com (September 4, 2003; September 4, 2003).

Schneiderman, A., M. Elbaum, T. Shultz, S. Keem, M. Greenebaum, and J. Driller. "Assessment of Dental Caries with Digital Imaging Fiber-Optic Transillumination (DIFOTI): In Vitro Study" (Abstract). cbi.nlm.nih.gov (1997; June 3, 2003).

Schneiderman, A., M. Elbaum, T. Schultz, S. Keem, M. Greenebaum, and J. Driller. "Assessment of Dental Caries with Digital Imaging Fiber-Optic Transillumination (DIFOTI™): In vitro Study." *Caries Research.* 1997; 31:130–110.

Smith, Kevin E. "Caries Detection: At Best an Inexact Science: Part II." *Global Dental Newsjournal.* global-dental.com (2000; June 3, 2003).

Stookey, George, and Carlos Gonzalez-Cabezas. "Emerging Methods of Caries Diagnosis." www.nidr.nih.gov (n.d.; June 2, 2003).

Urbankova, Alice, and Richard Lichtenthal. "DentSim Virtual Reality in Preclinical Operative Dentistry to Improve Psychomotor Skills: A Pilot Study." denx.com (2002; October 26, 2003).

White, Joel M., and W. Stephen Eakle. "Rationale and Treatment Approach in Minimally Invasive Dentistry." *JADA* 131 (June 2000): 13s–19s.

CHAPTER 7

Information Technology in Surgery

OUTLINE

- **Learning Objectives**
- **Overview**
- **Computer-Assisted Surgery**
  - *Computer-Assisted Surgical Planning*
  - *Minimally Invasive Surgery*
  - *Computer-Assisted Surgery and Robotics*
  - *ROBODOC, AESOP, ZEUS, da Vinci, MINERVA, and Other Robotic Devices*
  - *Augmented Reality*
  - *Telepresence Surgery*
  - *Discussion and Future Directions*
- **Lasers in Surgery**
- **Conclusion**
- **Selected Reading**
- **Chapter Summary**
- **Key Terms**
- **Review Questions**
  - *Multiple Choice*
  - *True/False Questions*
  - *Critical Thinking*
- **Sources**

LEARNING OBJECTIVES

Upon completion of this chapter, you will be able to

- List some of the uses of computers in surgery.
- Describe the role of computers in surgical planning.
- Define robot, endoscopic surgery, minimally invasive surgery, augmented reality, and telepresence surgery; be aware of the SOCRATES system that allows long distance mentoring of surgeons in real time.

- List some of the robots used in surgery including ROBODOC and AESOP, ZEUS and da Vinci.
- Describe some of the advantages and disadvantages of computer-assisted surgery.
- Describe the use of lasers in surgery.

OVERVIEW

Information technology is entering the twenty-first century with profound challenges and extraordinary techniques in the field of surgery. Hardware and software are being developed that help in the planning and implementation of surgical procedures. Sophisticated simulation software and speech recognition systems, in addition to **robots** equipped with **artificial intelligence**—programmed to "hear," "see," and "respond" to their environments, are already helping to perform certain operations. Special systems software is used to network all the computerized devices in an operating room.

Health care personnel can use a combination of computer-generated images, virtual and **augmented reality**, and robotic devices to assist prior to and during operations. Currently, computer-generated graphics assist in planning surgery, in guiding operations, and in training surgeons and other health care professionals. Enhanced images and precision instruments have made the development of the field of **minimally invasive surgery (MIS)** possible. MIS is surgery performed through small incisions. Most minimally invasive procedures are done using an **endoscope**—a thin tube that can be connected to a minuscule camera. It projects an image of the surgical site onto a monitor. The surgeon does not look at the patient; instead she or he looks at a monitor on which is projected an *image* of the patient. Thus, much **computer-assisted surgery** is said to be image-directed. **Distance** (or **telepresence**) **surgery** performed by robotic devices controlled by surgeons at another site has been successfully performed. It is conceivable that a robot controlled only by a computer program could perform surgery.

COMPUTER-ASSISTED SURGERY

Computer-Assisted Surgical Planning

Computer-assisted surgical planning involves the use of **virtual environment** technology to provide surgeons with realistic accurate models on which to teach surgery and plan and practice operations. With **virtual reality (VR)** technology, the computer can create an environment that seems real, but is not. Virtual reality simulations were first used in the 1940s to train pilots. Currently, these lifelike simulations are used in the health care field. The models created by VR technology can look, sound, and feel real. The models can respond to pressure by changing shape and to being cut by leaking. A model such as this, which is interactive, allows surgeons not only to plan surgeries more precisely, but also to practice operations without touching a patient. Some models include a predictive element, which shows the results of the doctor's actions. For example, plastic surgeons can practice on a model of a face and see the results of their work. The Netra system allows planning of biopsies, tumor resections, surgical implants, and surgery for motor disorders. The Compass system allows surgeons to plan operations for brain tumors by providing a three-dimensional model from CT scans and MRIs. The image is also used as a guide during the operation.

Minimally Invasive Surgery (MIS)

Minimally invasive surgery, utilizing an endoscope, performs procedures through small incisions that involve a minimum of damage to healthy tissue (Figure 7.1). There is less bleeding and pain and a shorter recovery time. This means a shorter

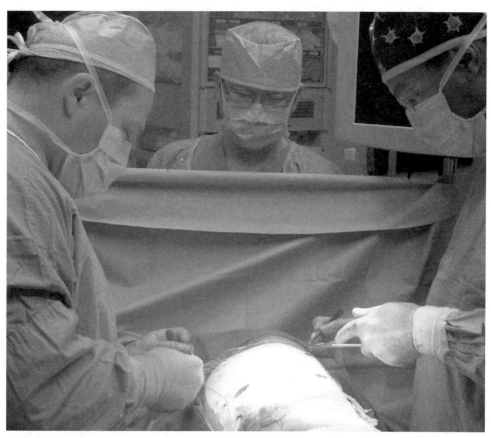

FIGURE 7.1 Miniature instruments and video cameras allow Drs. Robert Caccavale and Jean P. Bocage (left to right), thoracic surgeons at Saint Peter's University Hospital in New Brunswick, NJ, to perform minimally invasive thoracic surgery. Saint Peter's Video Assisted Thoracic Surgery (VATS) program offers patients a surgical option that is performed through two or three small incisions and results in a more comfortable and convenient recovery period.
Photo courtesy of Saint Peter's University Hospital, New Brunswick, NJ.

hospital stay and lower costs. You will recall that an endoscope projects an image of the surgical field onto a monitor. Recognizing that a picture on a monitor is not the same as viewing the surgical field, some doctors are attempting to improve the picture by connecting endoscopes to high-definition TVs. Gall bladder disease has been treated with minimally invasive techniques for many years.

Computer-Assisted Surgery and Robotics

Computer-assisted surgery makes use of robotics and computer-generated images such as CT scans and MRIs. The robots are under the control of software and the surgeon. Through a combination of hardware and software, a robot may be able to "see" via video devices and to "hear" through microphones using speech recognition software.

Robots, unlike humans, can hold endoscopes and other instruments without becoming tired or shaky. Robots are also used to scale down the surgeon's motions. Some surgeons report that this makes their hands "rock steady," making surgery on small delicate areas such as the eye safer.

Feedback mechanisms allow the robot to determine the proper pressure and tension needed to manipulate a particular object. Robots are able to compare tissue density and thus "decide" whether tissue is normal or a brain tumor by remembering the tissue's "pressure signature."

Currently, doctors are trying to give robots a delicate sense of touch; robots would be able to palpate tissue. To restore the sense of touch to surgeons, a chip containing 64 sensors would be inside the body; it would scan the patient. When it encountered a lump, the pressure in a sensor would rise. Outside the patient, the doctor's finger rests on motorized pins that rise/fall according to the sensors. Through the pins, the doctor will feel the object inside of the patient's body.

Currently robotics and MIS are being used in complex surgeries. New computer-controlled systems are making it possible to perform trauma surgery (such as femoral fracture fixation) through one-quarter-inch incisions; one such system has received FDA clearance. Minimally invasive knee and hip replacements are also a possibility. FDA-approved hardware and software will make hip replacement through a tiny incision possible. The software allows the surgeon to have more information by keeping track of the implant and the instruments and their relation to the patient. The information is given to the surgeon in real time.

New instruments are being developed to make surgery even less invasive. Laprotek is developing flexible, computer-controlled catheters capable of suturing; the surgeon can control them inside the patient. In May 2003, European clinical trials began.

One program, eXpert Trainer, attempts to teach the special skills that are needed to perform MIS. The skills include working with long instruments, learning "eye-hand disassociation" to work on a patient while looking at a monitor, working in a three-dimensional field while looking at a two-dimensional screen, and to reverse right and left motions and images.

ROBODOC, AESOP, ZEUS, da Vinci, MINERVA, and Other Robotic Devices

The earliest use of a robot in surgery was in hip replacement operations. Integrated Surgical Systems's **ROBODOC** (which is undergoing FDA-approved clinical trials) is a computer-controlled, image-directed robot that performed its first hip replacement in 1992. It can be used only with cementless implants—which constitute about one-third of those done each year. It has been used in thousands of hip replacement operations worldwide. Because ROBODOC actually cuts into a patient's femur, there have to be strict built-in safeguards. The safeguards come from the program that controls the robot and the physical limitations on how much ROBODOC can move. Prior to the operation, the Hip Navigation System helps surgeons align implants. The surgeon inserts three pins into the patient's hip. ROBODOC uses these as guides for locating the point to start drilling. Currently, some hip replacements are being performed without pins, and studies are being done comparing the two methods. ROBODOC works with ORTHODOC, which, using CT scans, creates a 3-D image of the hip. The doctor plans the surgery using the image. The plan is translated into drilling instructions for ROBODOC, which drills a perfect opening for the implant. ROBODOC is up to 10 times more accurate than a human being.

In a report of U.S. multicenter trials comparing outcomes of hip replacement done with ROBODOC to those performed by hand, it was found that at 24 months there were no differences in complications between the two groups; however, the group undergoing ROBODOC surgery had no intraoperative fractures even though blood loss and surgical time were greater. The most significant findings were that ROBODOC did "improve implant size, selection, position, and accuracy." One of the advantages of ROBODOC is that it forces surgeons to plan carefully, thus avoiding the wrong-sized implant and reaming defects. The study predicts better long-term performance with ROBODOC. A German study focused on safety. It found that an operation with ROBODOC had never had to be stopped for safety reasons. The robot itself would stop the surgery if it sensed any errors in data. It could then be completed by hand.

AESOP (Automated Endoscopic System for Optimal Positioning), which was introduced in 1994, by Computer Motion, Inc., is the first FDA-cleared surgical robot (Figure 7.2). Originally developed for the space program, AESOP is now used as an assistant in endoscopic procedures. It holds and moves the endoscope under the direction of the surgeon. AESOP was first developed to be controlled by foot pedals. However, currently it responds to voice commands such as "AESOP move left" or "AESOP stop." "AESOP move right" causes a continuous movement for 2.5 seconds. The surgeon can tell AESOP to save a position and to return to it later. Any surgeon who uses AESOP trains the robot to recognize his or her voice. If it fails to recognize the surgeon's voice or command during an operation, a backup system of manual controls can be used. Unlike a human assistant, AESOP does not become tired or shaky. It has been used in a wide variety of procedures, including appendectomy, splenectomy, and relief of intestinal obstruction.

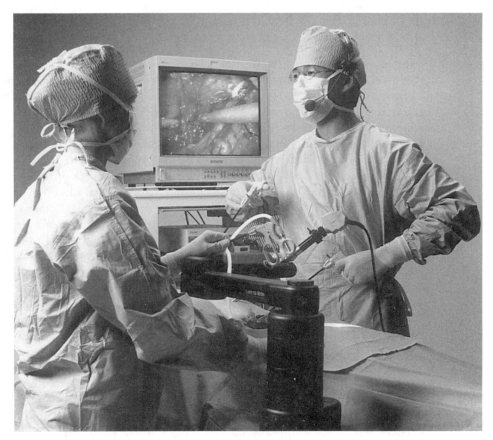

FIGURE 7.2   AESOP 3000, a voice-activated surgical robotic arm, holds the endoscope, providing a steady image.
Copyright Intuitive Surgical, Inc.

In May 1998, in France, heart surgery was performed on six patients using computers and robots. The incisions are small. The surgeon touches only the console located at a distance of several yards from the patient. She or he can see inside the heart via a three-dimensional camera inside the patient; the robot actually performs the surgery, directed by the surgeon. More and more cardiac surgeries are being performed as minimally invasive surgeries.

ZEUS is a robotic surgical system that will make minimally invasive microsurgery possible. ZEUS has three interactive robotic arms, one of which holds the endoscope, while the other two manipulate the surgical instruments. The surgeon, sitting at a console, controls them. The endoscope is controlled by voice commands. The surgeon manipulates instruments that resemble surgical tools while looking at a monitor. The surgeon's manipulations control the robotic arms, which are actually doing the surgery. ZEUS includes a feedback system so that the surgeon "feels" the tissue.

The computer-controlled robotic arms also scale down the surgeon's movements, filtering out any hand tremor. This means that a one-inch movement by the surgeon becomes a one-tenth of an inch movement of the robot's surgical instrument. By eliminating the hand's vibrations, ZEUS makes delicate procedures safer. Thus, ZEUS can increase the surgeon's dexterity. ZEUS can perform some heart bypass surgery endoscopically, through incisions the diameter of a pencil instead of the traditional 30-centimeter splitting of the breast bone. ZEUS may be approved for use in coronary bypass, mitral valve replacement, and laparoscopic and thoracic surgery.

Similar to ZEUS, the **da Vinci** system is also used for minimally invasive heart surgery. Da Vinci was first cleared for assisting in surgery in 1997, for performing some surgeries in 2000, and for performing cardiac surgery, such as mitral valve repair, in November 2002. A small study in December 2000 found that patients undergoing minimally invasive mitral valve repair had less pain and shorter hospital stays than those who had had conventional surgery. They return to work 50 percent faster. Minimally invasive heart surgeries are performed through three tiny incisions: One is for the endoscope that projects the surgical field on to a monitor; the other two are for the surgical instruments. The instruments are held by a robot. The robot's wrists can move 180 degrees (a greater range of motion than humans have) and follow the surgeon's hand motions; the surgeon's hands are attached to controls. The surgeon watches the surgery on a screen in three-dimensional, high-resolution images, and can see any part of the surgical field. One advantage of da Vinci is that it mimics the surgeon's hand motions. To control other laparoscopic instruments, the surgeon has to move the opposite way, for example, to move the instrument right, the surgeon must move left, up is down and so on. On January 17, 2002, the first endoscopic cardiac bypass surgery was performed in the United States. Da Vinci is also used to repair an inborn condition called atrial septal defect (ASD). Patients born with ASD have an opening between the two upper chambers of the heart, which, untreated, can result in congestive heart failure, hypertension, and increased risk of stroke.

It should be noted that at least one person has died in a robot-aided surgery. Da Vinci was being used to remove a cancerous kidney. However, the patient's aorta was accidentally cut during the surgery, and he died two days later. The hospital denied that the robot was to blame.

MINERVA is a robot developed to perform stereotactic neurosurgical procedures. Used to treat some brain tumors, the stereotactic method involves fixing a metal frame, similar to a cage, on the patient's head. The surgeon uses an MRI or CT scan to calculate how to reach the tumor with a minimum of trauma to surrounding tissue. The surgeon does not see the surgical site and must rely on the CT scan to avoid damaging vital parts of the brain. For successful robot-assisted surgery, the robot must be highly accurate. MINERVA would operate inside the CT scan. This enables the surgeon to follow the position of the instruments. The doctor selects the target. MINERVA does the calculations, and responding to the doctor's commands, performs the procedure. NeuroMate was developed in France for neurosurgical applications and is FDA approved. It has performed over 1,000 tumor biopsies. It collects data from images of the patient and with special software plans the path to the tumor. This information is transferred to a control workstation. The surgeon uses all the information including X-rays to command the robot to insert a guide. The guide is then used to introduce a surgical instrument. Less invasive than robot-assisted stereotactic neurosurgery is stereotactic radiosurgery, or gamma knife surgery (see chapter 5 on Radiology), which does not involve cutting but uses radiation to shrink certain brain tumors that then may not need to be surgically removed.

Other robots have been developed. Using **ARTEMIS**, a surgical system that works with the simulation software **KISMET**, a surgeon can perform MIS while viewing three screens, which show the view presented by the endoscope and simulations. ARTEMIS can also perform minimally invasive breast biopsies.

Robots can assist in needle placement in the insertion of nerve blocks for back pain and minimally invasive kidney procedures (PAKY/RCM—percutaneous access of the kidney/remote center of motion). Acrobat (active constraint robot) is used for total knee replacement. Probot helps in prostate surgery. Steady-Hand robot was developed for microsurgery, where smaller than human movements of the hand are needed. A robot is being developed in Germany, which reduces the risks of extremely delicate spinal surgery; it would make it possible to monitor the surgery in real time, possibly diminishing risks such as paralysis.

System software is required to connect the operating room hardware into a network that a surgeon can control with voice commands. **HERMES** is an FDA-cleared operating system that performs these tasks, allowing the surgeon to use his or her voice to control all the electronic equipment in the operating room, coordinating the endoscope and robotic devices. It also allows the surgeon to adjust lighting with a voice command. The surgeon can use HERMES to take and print pictures and access the patient's electronic medical record, including images and other information.

Augmented Reality

Because much computer-assisted surgery is image guided, software has been developed that enhances what the surgeon sees. This kind of surgery is called augmented reality surgery. It makes use of computer-generated imagery to provide the surgeon with information that would otherwise be unavailable. The computer-generated images may either be fused with the image on the monitor or projected directly onto the patient's body during the operation, allowing the doctor to virtually see inside the patient. However, an image on a monitor is two-dimensional. A head mounted display, which combines the computer-generated images and the image of the patient, allows the surgeon to see a three-dimensional field and see different views by simply turning her or his head instead of adjusting the endoscope, making it more like traditional open surgery. The image and the reality must of course be perfectly aligned (registered) with each other. One use of augmented reality is in using an ultrasound to allow the technician to see an image of the fetus on the abdomen of the patient. Another is in image-guided breast biopsies. It is also used in brain surgery, where an MRI or CT scan may be projected on the patient's head, so that the surgeon can see a tumor that otherwise would be invisible.

Telepresence Surgery

Telepresence surgery (distance surgery) is at the cutting edge of telemedicine. NASA first sought to develop telepresence surgery for space flight medical emergencies. Actual surgeries have been performed with the patient and surgeon at a distance and have been successful. Distance surgery thus has the potential of making surgical expertise available on battlefields, space stations, and in remote rural areas. Several research groups are working on telesurgical systems. Some of this work is funded by the Advanced Research Projects Agency (ARPA) of the U.S. Department of Defense, which first conceived of robotic surgery and which still sees remote surgery as a way of saving lives on the battlefield and protecting surgeons from dangerous environments. One of the systems that has been developed is the Green Telepresence Surgical System, in which surgeons wearing three-dimensional glasses can view the operating room and patient. The system has been used to practice suturing. It has demonstrated its precision by slicing a grape into one-millimeter slices. Distance operations were first performed on animals.

In telepresence surgery, as in MIS, the doctor looks at an *image* of the patient, not the actual patient. The instruments in the surgeon's hands feel real, but in fact only direct the robot at a distant site (theoretically hundreds of miles away), which is actually performing the surgery.

In September 2001, a woman in France had her gall bladder removed by doctors in New York. She spent two days in the hospital. Technically, the surgery made use of high-speed fiber optics, so that time delay was minimal. Much of the system is not yet FDA approved. "It was amazing for the doctors . . . to see the surgical tools suddenly start moving themselves and doing the operation, without any surgeon in the room guiding them," according to one of the doctors on the French team (Klarreich, 2001). In this computer-assisted laparoscopic procedure patient and doctor never touch; the surgeon controls the robot through hand signals. Successful prostate cancer surgery was performed in April 2002, between Germany and Virginia. Using the **SOCRATES** system, the American doctor was able to see and hear as if he were in the operating room in Berlin; he also controlled AESOP while the German surgeon did the surgery. Using SOCRATES, the remote doctor can teleconnect to the operating room, see and hear, and control devices networked by HERMES. SOCRATES is basically a mentoring system, allowing a surgeon in one place to give expert advice in real-time to a distant surgeon. In 2001 the SOCRATES system was cleared by the FDA, which at the same time created a new classification of device: Robotic Telemedicine Device.

In March 2003, ZEUS was used to perform distance surgery in Canada to correct a patient's acid reflux disease. At one hospital, endoscopic instruments were inserted into the patient's stomach. At another hospital 400 kilometers away a surgeon used ZEUS to perform the successful surgery. ZEUS's sensors took the information from the surgeon's hand movements and sent it to the distant instruments. The Canadian federal government sees distance surgery as a way of serving its northern population.

Discussion and Future Directions

Computer-assisted surgery encompasses everything from the well-established use of a robotic assistant in an endoscopic procedure to telepresence surgery. It is an evolving field. New robotic devices, new software, new techniques, and new applications are being developed. Thus, this cannot be an exhaustive survey of the uses of robotics, augmented reality techniques, or minimally invasive surgical procedures. Currently, computer-generated images help make surgery more precise. MIS results in smaller incisions, less trauma, and therefore less pain and shorter recovery time. This leads to some economic benefits, including shorter hospitals stays and less time lost from work. Even though the equipment is quite expensive, it may be less expensive in the long run to use a robot than a human assistant to hold an endoscope in the operating room. However, there are substantial difficulties involved in using MIS. The workspace is small. The doctor is looking at a monitor, not a patient while *indirectly* manipulating surgical instruments. This may cause the surgeon to be less dexterous and have less eye-hand coordination. Research is currently being done to help solve these problems. A glovelike device is being developed to help the surgeon control minimally invasive tools more easily.

LASERS IN SURGERY

Laser stands for light amplification by the stimulated emission of radiation. Each type of laser produces a different wavelength of light. Lasers can cut, vaporize tissue and tumors, and seal small blood vessels. There are advantages to using lasers in surgery. A laser beam can be narrowed to the size of a few cells. Using lasers, a doctor can reach places that traditional surgery cannot touch. Because lasers coagulate blood, bleeding is minimized. The lasers' precision leads to faster healing and may make the actual surgery less painful.

Currently lasers are used in a variety of specialties including gynecology, orthopedics, urology, ear, nose, and throat, cardiovascular, and gastroenterology. Lasers are used in patients with angina (severe chest pain) to make small channels through the heart muscle. This decreases pain. Lasers are also used to destroy cancer cells in esophageal and some lung cancers.

LASIK is eye surgery involving lasers. Its purpose is to correct vision, so that patients are less dependent on glasses. After cutting a flap in the cornea using a knife, the laser produces a beam of ultraviolet light which is used to vaporize the middle part of the cornea. The laser used is a cold laser, which does not hurt surrounding tissue. This procedure changes the shape of the cornea permanently, reducing or eliminating the need for glasses.

CONCLUSION

Computer-assisted surgery holds great promise for the future. The use of augmented images to teach surgeons and plan and guide operations can reduce unnecessary cutting and make operations more precise and less invasive. This chapter highlighted many of the benefits of minimally invasive procedures and the use of robots. However, it should be remembered that aside from a few established procedures such as cementless hip replacement and gall bladder removal, this field is in its infancy. It is also important to keep in mind the dangers and disadvantages. Looking at a monitor is never quite as good as looking at a live patient; feeling via sensory feedback mechanisms is not the same as actually having one's hands on living tissue. MIS is more difficult to learn and requires more training than traditional surgery. Further, doctors trained in traditional open surgery methods will be understandably reluctant to learn the new methods.

The most experimental area of computer-assisted surgery is telepresence or distance surgery. High-bandwidth channels are required for transmission, and networks must be 100% reliable, since any delay or failure could result in the death of a patient. At the present time, the Canadian federal government is working with doctors to promote the use of distance surgery to treat rural populations.

SELECTED READING

Meadows, Michelle. "Robots Lend a Helping Hand to Surgeons." *FDA Consumer.* www.fda.gov (May–June 2002; June 16, 2003).

IN THE NEWS

Robots Lend a Helping Hand to Surgeons

by Michelle Meadows

Robot-assisted surgery is the latest development in the larger movement of endoscopy, a type of minimally invasive surgery—the idea being that less invasive procedures translate into less trauma and pain for patients. Surgery through smaller incisions typically results in less scarring and faster recovery. It's not that robots are changing the basics of surgery. Surgeons are still cutting and sewing like they have been for decades. Robots represent a new computer-assisted tool that provides another way for surgeons to work.

Rather than cutting patients open, endoscopy allows surgeons to operate through small incisions by using an endoscope. This fiber optic instrument has a small video camera that gives doctors a magnified internal view of a surgical site on a television screen.

In abdominal endoscopy, known as laparoscopy, surgeons thread the fiber optic instrument into the abdomen. First performed in the late 1980s, laparoscopy is now routine for many procedures, such as surgery on the gallbladder and on female organs.

Robots Lend a Helping Hand to Surgeons *(continued)*

With robotic surgical systems, surgeons don't move endoscopic instruments directly with their hands. Instead, surgeons sit at a console several feet from the operating table and use joysticks similar to those used in video games. They perform surgical tasks by guiding the movement of the robotic arms in a process known as tele-manipulation.

The Food and Drug Administration reviews data on the safety and effectiveness of robotic software and hardware and requires manufacturers to implement training programs for surgeons. The FDA also monitors experimental uses for robotic applications, including clinical trials for robotic heart surgery. It's too soon to say for sure how far and how fast robotic surgery will grow, but experts say the future looks promising.

Robotics and Telesurgery

The da Vinci and ZEUS make it possible for surgeons to perform robotic surgery across long distances. Surgeons from the European Institute of Technology used ZEUS and high-speed telecommunications to perform the first complete long-distance robotic surgery last year. According to an article in the September 27, 2001, issue of the journal *Nature,* the surgeons worked from New York to remove the gallbladder of a 68-year-old woman in Strasbourg, France.

The mean total time delay was 155 milliseconds, so surgeons could see the result of their commands a little more than one-tenth of a second later. The time to set up the robot was 16 minutes and the gallbladder was dissected in 54 minutes without complications. This is similar to the time it takes to perform standard laparoscopic gallbladder surgery. Mount Sinai Medical Center in New York and the Department of Electrical Engineering at the University of California participated in the study. Researchers first practiced the procedure on pigs.

CHAPTER SUMMARY

This chapter introduced the student to some of the uses of information technology in surgery.

- Computer-assisted surgery involves the use of computer technology in the planning and/or performance of operations.
- Computer-generated images make planning operations more precise and allow surgeons to practice on realistic models.
- In the operating room, robotic devices that can "see," "hear," and respond are used as surgical assistants.
  - Robotic devices are used in minimally invasive surgery, much of which involves the use of an endoscope, a viewing device, which can project an image of the surgical site onto a monitor. The image is used to guide the surgeon.

- ROBODOC, AESOP, ZEUS, da Vinci, and MINERVA are robots used in minimally invasive endoscopic procedures.
- In MIS, 3-D computer-generated images may be fused with the image of the surgical site or actually projected onto the patient to enhance or augment reality.
- The surgeon's manipulations guide the robotic arms, which operate on the patient. Voice commands control the arm that holds the endoscope.
- Telepresence surgery, in which the surgeon is at one site and the patient at another site, is being performed. The SOCRATES system allows a surgeon to mentor another surgeon at a distant location in real time.
- Lasers are used in a variety of specialties.

KEY TERMS

AESOP
ARTEMIS
artificial intelligence
augmented reality
  (enhanced reality)
computer-assisted surgery
da Vinci
distance surgery (tele-
  presence surgery)

endoscope
HERMES
KISMET
laparoscope
laser
LASIK
MINERVA
minimally invasive
  surgery (MIS)

ROBODOC
robots
telepresence surgery
  (distance surgery)
SOCRATES
virtual environment
virtual reality (VR)
ZEUS

REVIEW QUESTIONS

Multiple Choice

1. A robot _____.
   A. Can respond to speech commands
   B. Is a programmable machine
   C. A and B
   D. None of the above
2. _____ may be used to help train surgeons and to allow realistic practice operations.
   A. Virtual environment technology
   B. Endoscopes
   C. Robots
   D. ZEUS
3. _____ is a robotic device used in some hip replacement operations.
   A. ROBODOC
   B. AESOP
   C. ZEUS
   D. HERMES

4. An endoscope is _____.
   A. A surgical instrument that cuts into the patient
   B. Only used to produce the image the surgeon sees
   C. A thin tube with a light source
   D. B and C
5. Surgery that makes use of computer-generated images to enhance what the surgeon sees is called _____.
   A. Virtual reality
   B. Augmented reality
   C. Telepresence surgery
   D. None of the above
6. Among the benefits of MIS are _____.
   A. Smaller scars
   B. Shorter recovery time
   C. Less trauma to healthy tissue
   D. All of the above
7. The most frequently done laparoscopic procedure is _____.
   A. Gall bladder removal
   B. Open heart surgery
   C. Brain surgery
   D. Knee replacement
8. The first FDA-cleared surgical robot was _____.
   A. ZEUS
   B. HERMES
   C. AESOP
   D. HARRY
9. Computer technology may be involved in _____.
   A. Planning operations
   B. Assisting in the operating room
   C. Training surgeons
   D. All of the above
10. A robot developed to assist in brain surgery is _____.
    A. ZEUS
    B. HERMES
    C. AESOP
    D. MINERVA

True/False Questions

1. The high-bandwidth communications lines needed for distance surgery are in place. _____
2. Computer-generated graphics can virtually give a surgeon X-ray vision. _____
3. One of the advantages of MIS is that the surgeon looks at a monitor not at the patient. _____
4. A robotic device can "decide" whether what it is touching is a tumor or normal tissue. _____

5. Telepresence surgery was first conceived of by the U.S. Department of Defense. _____
6. A disadvantage of MIS is longer hospital stays. _____
7. Virtual reality technology creates environments that seem real but are not. _____
8. Surgeons make use of computer models to plan operations. _____
9. Some surgical robots were originally developed for the space program. _____
10. Hip replacement operations using ROBODOC cannot possibly be as good as those with human surgeons only. _____

Critical Thinking

1. Many challenging issues arise from the innovative uses of computer-assisted surgery and the use of robots in the operating room. (a) Discuss how these developments might affect the patient and the surgeon. (b) What do you consider the responsibilities of the hardware manufacturer? (c) What do you consider the responsibilities of the software publisher?
2. Discuss the advantages and disadvantages of robotic surgery to the patient and the surgeon.
3. Given that computers are playing a more active role in surgery, what steps would you recommend be taken to protect patients from the effects of computer viruses, electrical malfunctions, and software bugs?
4. "Imagine you're having a hip replacement. . . . As you're wheeled into the operating room, you notice the nurses and anesthetist preparing for your surgery. But wait, someone's missing. Your surgeon. You look around the room and finally spot the surgeon, off in the corner keying information into a computer terminal. And there, next to the doctor and the computer, is a 500-pound, seven-foot-high, jointed steel arm, with a tiny drill attached to one end. It's ROBODOC. And it's going to assist in your surgery" (Ropp, 1993). How do you feel about being operated on by a robot as opposed to a human being?

SOURCES

"About Lasers in Medicine." http://www.abbottnorthwestern.com (January 29, 2004; January 29, 2004).

Ackerman, Jeremy. "Ultrasound Visualization Research." cs.unc.edu (June 15, 2000; June 6, 2003).

Argenziano, Michael. "Robotically Assisted, Minimally Invasive Cardiac Surgery." http://columbiasurgery.org (March 12, 2002; June 5, 2003).

"Artemis Medical Receives 510K Clearance on New Image Guided Biopsy Device." Artemismedical.com (April 22, 2002; June 7, 2003).

Bargar, William L., Jeffery K. Taylor, Roderick H. Turner, Joseph C. McCarthy, Anthony M. DiGioia, III, and Dana C. Mears. "ROBODOC multicenter trial: An Interim Report." Americam Academy of Orthopedic Surgeons 1996 Annual Meeting—Scientific Program, New Orleans. www.aaos.org (1996; June 7, 2003).

Cleary, Kevin, and Charles, Nguyen. "State of the Art in Surgical Robotics: Clinical Applications and Technology Challenges." 141.161.165.150/publications/State of the Art Surgical Robotics.pdf (February 24, 2002; June 7, 2003).

"Computer Assisted Total Hip Replacement Surgery." smith-nephew.com (n.d.; June 4, 2003).

"Computer Assisted Total Knee Replacement Surgery." smith-nephew.com (n.d.; June 4, 2003).

"Dr. Argensiano Reports Shorter Hospital Stay, Improved Recovery Time with Robotically Assisted Heart Surgery." columbiasurgery.org (November 2002; June 5, 2003).

Eisenberg, Anne. "What's Next; Restoring the Human Touch to Remote-Controlled Surgery." nyt.com (January 24, 2002; October 12, 2003).

———. "What's Next; A Sharper Picture of What Ails the Body." nyt.com (January 24, 2002; October 11, 2003).

Elliott, Victoria Stagg. "New Surgical Technology: Dr. Roboto." amednews.com (November 20, 2000; June 8, 2003).

ENDOVIA Medical Commences Human Clinical Trials. endoviamedical.com (May 8, 2003; June 4, 2003).

"Evolution of Minimally Invasive and Robotic Cardiac Surgery." columbiasurgery.org (n.d. but after 2000; June 5, 2003).

"eXpert Trainer." hmc.psu.edu (September 9, 2003; October 13, 2003).

"FDA Approves First Robot for Surgery." www.intuisurg.com, (August 23, 2000; June 8, 2003).

"FDA Clearance of da Vinci Surgical System for Intracardiac Surgery Now Encompasses 'ASD' Closure." www.intuisurg.com (January 30, 2003; June 5, 2003).

"Florida Man Dies after Surgery Involving Robotic Device." Injuryboard.com (October 31, 2002; June 8, 2003).

Hall, Alan. "Computer Surgeons Make the Cut," http://www.businessweek.com, (June 14, 2001; June 9, 2003).

"How the da Vinci Surgical System Works." columbiasurgery.org (2002; June 5, 2003).

"It's Your Health." Health Canada, Laser Eye Surgery. http://www.hc-sc.gc.ca/english/iyh/medical/laser_eye.html (November 18, 2002; February 2, 2004).

Junnarkar, Sandeep. "Virtual Reality Guides Surgeon's Hands." *New York Times Cybertimes.* http://www.nytimes.com (October 25, 1996; May 30, 1999).

Klarreich, Erica. "Is There a Doctor on the Planet?" nature.com (September 19, 2001; October 17, 2003).

Landers, Susan J. "Surgery from Six Feet Away: Robot Technology Becomes OR Reality." amednews.com (February 11, 2002; June 8, 2003).

LASIK Eye Surgery, U.S. Food and Drug Administration. www.FDA.gov (January 7, 2004; January 14, 2004).

Livingston, Mark. "UNC Laparoscopic Visualization Research." cs.unc.edu (August 11, 1998; June 6, 2003).

"Long-Distance Surgery Ushers in a 'New Era in Telehealth'." Betterhumans Staff. betterhumans.com (March 5, 2003; August 15, 2003).

Mack, Michael J. "Minimally Invasive and Robotic Surgery" *JAMA* 285 (February 7, 2001).

Meadows, Michelle. "Robots Lend a Helping Hand to Surgeons." *FDA Consumer.* www.fda.gov (May–June 2002; June 16, 2003).

"Medical Robotics @ UC Berkeley." robotics.eecs.Berkeley.edu (January 2002; June 6, 2003).

"Minimally Invasive Surgery." UPMC www.upmc.edu (2001; June 6, 2003).

"New Generation of Computer-Guided Endoscopic Instruments." endoviamedical.com (August 29, 2002; June 4, 2003).

"New York Weill Cornell Performs among First Minimally Invasive Kidney Removals in Children and Infants in New York." http://www.nycornell.org/news/press/kidney1.html (March 8, 2000; June 8, 2003).

Peterson, Lynne. "Trends-in-Medicine." trends-in-medicine.com (February 2003; June 5, 2003).

"Primary and Revision Total Hip Replacement Using Robodoc" (originally published in *Clinical Orthopaedics and Related Research*). jointsurgeons.com (2002; June 6, 2003).

"Redefining Surgery." robodoc.com (January 2002; June 6, 2003).

"Remote Control Telemedicine: Sponsored by the National Institutes of Health." http://www.ngi.gov/apps/nih/rem.html (n.d.; June 16, 2003).

"Revolutionizing Trauma Surgery." smith-nephew.com (n.d. but after 2001; June 4, 2003).

"Robot Reduces Spinal Injury Risk." news.bbc.co.uk (March 12, 2000; June 8, 2003).

"Robotic Surgical Assistant for Brain Surgery." NASA Space Telerobotic program. http://ranier.hq.nasa.gov/telerobotics (May 10, 1996; June 16, 2003).

"Robots." *Star-Ledger,* June 8, 1997, pp. 1, 12.

Ropp, Kevin L. "Robots in the Operating Room." *FDA Consumer* (July/August 1993; reprinted in 2002). http://www.fda.gov/bbs/topics/CONSUMER/CON00242.html.

Schaaf, Tracy, "Robotic Surgery: The Future Is Now." devicelink.com (2001; October 14, 2003).

Schurr, M. O., G. Buess, B. Neisius, and U. Voges. "Robotics and Telemanipulation Technologies for Endoscopic Surgeries: A Review of the ARTEMIS Project" (Abstract). ncbi.nlm.nih.gov (April 2000; October 14, 2003).

"Smith and Nephew Enhanced Hip Surgery with Highly Accurate Computer-Assisted Navigation." smith-nephew.com, (January 2, 2003; June 4, 2003).

"Smith and Nephew Launches Minimally Invasive Computer-Assisted Trauma Instruments." smith-nephew.com, (December 5, 2002; June 4, 2003).

Third Annual Meeting of the International Society for Computer Assisted Orthopaedic Surgery. www.caos-international.org/spage32.htm (June 18–21, 2003; October 18, 2003).

Vase, Ajit, "Robotic Laparoscopic Surgery: A Comparison of the da Vinci and ZEUS Systems." http://www.bhj.org/journal/2002_4402_apr/endo_208.htm (2002; October 15, 2003).

Versweyveld, Leslie. "Socrates Surgical Mentor Allows Surgeon Experts to Provide Remote Guidance in Complex Procedures." *Virtual Medical Worlds.* hoise.com (March 8, 2001; June 5, 2003).

———. "Thoroscopic Surgery Robots Now FDA-Approved for Use in United States Hospitals." *Virtual Medical Worlds.* hoise.com (March 6, 2001; June 5, 2003).

———. "US Food and Drug Administration Kept Busy Approving Surgical Robots from Various Market Competitors." *Virtual Medical Worlds.* hoise.com (October 17, 2001; June 5, 2003).

"Virtual Environments for Surgical Training and Augmentation." eecs.Berkeley.edu (February 27, 2001; June 6, 2003).

CHAPTER 8

Information Technology in Pharmacy

OUTLINE

- **Learning Objectives**
- **Overview**
- **Biotechnology and the Human Genome Project**
  - *Rational Drug Design*
  - *Bioinformatics*
  - *The Human Genome Project*
  - *Developments in Biotechnology*
- **Computer-Assisted Drug Trials**
- **Computer-Assisted Drug Review**
- **The Computerized Pharmacy**
  - *Computers and Drug Errors*
  - *The Automated Community Pharmacy*
  - *Automating the Hospital Pharmacy*
  - *The Hospital Pharmacy Robot and Bar Codes*
  - *Point-of-Use Drug Dispensing*
- **Telepharmacy**
- **Drug Delivery on a Chip**
- **The Impact of Information Technology on Pharmacy**
- **Selected Reading**
- **Chapter Summary**
- **Key Terms**
- **Review Questions**
  - *Multiple Choice*
  - *True/False Questions*
  - *Critical Thinking*
- **Sources**

LEARNING OBJECTIVES

Upon completion of this chapter, you will be able to

- Describe the contributions of information technology to the development and testing of drugs.
- Define biotechnology and rational drug design.
- Discuss the significance of the Human Genome Project and its contribution to the understanding of genetic diseases.
- List the uses of computers in clinical drug trials.
- Discuss the relationship of the understanding of the molecular basis of a disease to real breakthroughs in treatment.
- List the uses of computer technology in pharmacies, including
  - The use of computers in the neighborhood drug store, from the printing of drug information for customers to the full automation of the process of filling prescriptions using robots and bar codes
    - The use of computers in hospital pharmacies
      - In centralized dispensing systems using robots and bar codes
      - In decentralized point-of-use dispensing units
- Discuss telepharmacy, that is, the linking of pharmacists via telecommunications lines to dispensing units in remote locations such as doctors' offices.
- Discuss the impact of information technology on pharmacy as it affects pharmacists, patients, and hospital administrators.

OVERVIEW

Information technology is transforming all aspects of pharmacy from the design, testing, and approval of drugs to the automation of drug stores in the community, to the automation of hospital pharmacies and drug delivery systems. Telepharmacy, or the linking of the prescribing doctor's office with the dispensing pharmacy via telecommunications lines, is expanding.

BIOTECHNOLOGY AND THE HUMAN GENOME PROJECT

Rational Drug Design

The technical details of drug design are beyond the scope of this text. However, computers are being used to help design and test new drugs. **Biotechnology** sees the human body as a collection of molecules, and seeks to understand and treat disease in terms of these molecules. It attempts to identify the molecule causing a problem and then create another to correct it. Specific drugs are aimed at inhibiting the work of a specific disease-causing agent. In order to be effective, the drug needs to bind to its target molecule. It needs to fit, something like a key in a lock. To achieve an exact fit, the precise structure of the target must be mapped. Powerful computers allow scientists to create graphical models. Before the availability of computer technology, many drugs were discovered by accident or trial and error. One way of developing drugs with the help of computers is called **rational drug design**. Developing drugs by design requires mapping the structure and creating a three-dimensional graphical model of the target molecule. Since this involves a huge number of mathematical calculations, without computers the process took many years; after the calculations were completed, a wire model of the molecule had to be constructed. Now, supercomputers accurately do the calculations in a small fraction of the time, and graphical software produces the image on a computer screen. This is an example of the field of **scientific visualization**, which is defined by Donna Cox of the National Center for Supercomputing Applications as the process of graphically representing the results of numerical calculations. The model can be manipulated, rotated, and viewed from any angle. Specialized software is used to evaluate a drug's molecular structure, which can then be chemically synthesized. Of course, any compound developed this way still has to be tested in a *real* biological system. The modeling of the target molecule and development of the drug can be repeated several times until a chemical compound is found that satisfactorily inhibits or stimulates the activity of the target site's receptors. Drugs, that are used for Alzheimer's, hypertension, and AIDS have been developed with the help of computers.

Bioinformatics

The application of information technology to biology is called **bioinformatics**. This field seeks to organize biological data into databases. The information is then available to researchers who can search through existing data and add new entries of their own. These databases are made possible by the Human Genome Project.

The Human Genome Project

The development of new medications is becoming more dependent on knowledge of genes. The **Human Genome Project** (HGP), sponsored in the United States by the National Institutes of Health and the Department of Energy, began in 1990 and involved hundreds of scientists all over the world. It was "an . . . effort to understand the hereditary instructions that make each of us unique. The goal is to find the location of the 100,000 or so human genes and to read the entire genetic script, all three billion bits of information, by the year 2005." The project has succeeded in mapping the human genome. One of its goals is an attempt to understand the molecular bases of genetic diseases. This project would be inconceivable without computers and the Internet. Computers are used to keep track of the genes as they are identified; this prevents duplication of effort and ensures that no genes are overlooked. The Internet allows findings to be immediately communicated to scientists working on the project anywhere in the world. Three to four thousand diseases are caused by errors in genes. Altered genes also contribute to the development of other disorders such as cancer, heart disease, and diabetes. The Human Genome Project

expects to be able to identify such genes, which might make prevention, early detection, and treatment possible. Once the gene is identified, drugs can be designed.
Treatment may include gene therapy to replace the defective gene or the development of drugs. Ultimately, gene therapy may be tailored to specific patients. It should
be noted, however, that as of September 2003, few disease-related genes had been
identified, and that the identification of a disease-related gene is simply a starting
point for research. For example, one of the genes related to stroke was identified in
2003, but according to Dr. Jonathan Rosand, a stroke specialist at Massachusetts
General Hospital, it "is unlikely to yield new treatments any time soon" (Wade, 2003).

More than 25 million Americans suffer from rare and genetic diseases. The
Genetic and Rare Diseases Information Center, using information gathered by the
HGP, provides health care consumers with reliable, immediate, and free information. In one 3-month period, the Center received 1,000 calls and e-mails asking for
information ("Center to Offer Quick, Reliable Source for Genetic Information," n.d.).

The Human Genome Project is the basis for new databases of biological information. Computers are being used to quickly screen tens of thousands of compounds
a day, databases of genes, to find codes that could be useful in drug development.
Then a model can be constructed and a drug rationally designed. It is a new form of
trial and error, accelerated by computers, producing enormous amounts of information for researchers and computers to analyze.

Developments in Biotechnology

Understanding the molecular basis of a disease can lead to medical advances. In
September 1998, the U.S. **Food and Drug Administration (FDA)** approved Herceptin
as effective against certain types of metastatic breast cancer. Herceptin can work for
patients who have too much of a specific gene in their tumor cells. The gene (HER-
2/neu) produces a protein that engenders growth in the tumor cells. Herceptin
binds to this protein and inhibits its work. According to Dr. Dennis Slamon, who directed the research, the development of Herceptin "proves . . . that if we understand
what is broken in the malignant cell, we may be able to fix it." Herceptin may also to
be effective in fighting other cancers, including gastric, endometrial, pancreatic,
prostate, and colorectal cancers. Many other drugs are in the testing stages.

Clinical trials for Lucentis for the treatment of macular degeneration continue
in 2003. Lucentis is an antibody that binds to a protein that is involved in the
formation of blood vessels. In an early study, it was found that patients given
Lucentis on the average either maintained or gained vision, while the patients who
did not take Lucentis but received traditional treatments experienced an average
loss of vision.

In 2003, the FDA approved fast track status for the development, testing, and
review of Avastin, an antibody that inhibits the protein that plays a role in the maintenance and metastases of tumors. The protein, called vascular endothelial growth
factor (VEGF), helps in the creation of new blood vessels for the tumor. The protein is active in cancers, including metastatic colorectal, kidney, breast, and
non–small lung cancers. The most extensive trials have been with patients with

metastatic colorectal cancer. However, Avastin is also being tested on more than 20 different kinds of tumors.

In 2003, the FDA granted orphan drug status—a legal status meant to encourage the development of treatments for rare conditions—to Tarceva. Tarceva is designed for patients with a rare form of brain cancer. It targets a growth pathway in the cell and inhibits its activity, thus stopping the growth of the tumor. It is also being tested for use against advanced pancreatic cancer.

In 2003 the FDA approved the use of Xolair as a treatment for asthma. Xolair binds to IgE antibodies in the blood, which may trigger asthmatic symptoms. This decreases the release of chemicals that lead to the symptoms.

Antisense technology is one experimental technology used to develop drugs to shut off disease-causing genes. It has not been very successful. In a large clinical trial of a drug called Genasense, the results were mixed. Genasense promised to enhance chemotherapy in cancer patients by shutting off the gene producing bcl-2, which helps cells stay alive. However, in a trial on 771 patients, it extended the lives of patients less than two months, which is not statistically significant; it did, however, shrink tumors in 12 percent as compared with 7 percent in the control group.

Another new technology aimed at drug development is called **RNA interference** or **RNAi**. RNA stands for ribonucleic acid. It is made in the nucleus of a cell, but is not restricted to the nucleus. It is a long, coiled-up molecule whose purpose is to take the blueprint from DNA and build our actual proteins. RNAi is a process that cells use to turn off genes. The attempt at developing drugs based on RNAi is in its infancy, and would, if successful, turn off genes associated with disease. Prior attempts at turning off genes with drugs have not succeeded.

COMPUTER-ASSISTED DRUG TRIALS

Before a drug can be marketed, it has to undergo extensive clinical trials. Some last as long as six years and cost over $100 million. Now, however, software has been developed that allows companies to simulate clinical trials on a computer before the actual trials begin. A simulated drug trial uses information about the drug's effects from earlier trials, animal studies, or trials of similar drugs. By trying out many "what ifs" on computer models, the actual trials can be more precisely designed, making it more likely that they will be definitive. Critics maintain that the models are not precise enough because knowledge of the human body is incomplete. The **Physiome Project** has created a virtual heart using mathematical equations to simulate the processes of the heart. It has been used in studies of irregular heartbeats. The project is developing a virtual body on which to test drugs, and will then attempt to create a virtual immune system to find treatments for conditions such as arthritis and autoimmune disorders. These mathematical models will help reduce the time necessary to test drugs. However, computer-assisted drug trials are not a replacement for actual clinical trials; they are a tool to make the actual trials more effective. The purpose of **computer-assisted trial design (CATD)** is to decrease the time and money spent on the trial phase of drug development.

COMPUTER-ASSISTED DRUG REVIEW

After a new drug has been developed, the Food and Drug Administration reviews it. In 1995, the FDA began computerizing the drug review and approval process. This enables them to speed up the process by reviewing data online. According to the *FDA Consumer,* what used to take weeks can now be done in an instant. With FDA computers networked to a drug company's computer, data from clinical trials can be transferred instantly and reviewed more quickly than in the past. It is also easier to do comparisons with other drugs and spot possible problems. According to Roger Williams, of the FDA's Center for Drug Evaluation, the drug review process makes use of giant electronic spreadsheets of perhaps 300 million cells for each review area for each drug. Computers make it possible to organize this massive amount of data.

THE COMPUTERIZED PHARMACY

Computers were introduced in pharmacies more than 20 years ago. Initially, drug orders in hospitals could be entered into a computer. The computer system checked for adverse drug interactions and specific patient drug allergies. Today, computers can maintain complete medication profiles of all patients on databases, and warn of drug interactions and allergies. This use of the database not only protects patients, but also makes information more easily available for national and international drug studies.

Computers and Drug Errors

Computerizing any aspect of prescription entry, the filling of orders, and dispensing of medications appears to lead to a decrease in medication errors. Currently, computers are utilized in both hospital pharmacies and community drug stores. In any corner drug store, computers provide drug information for patients. According to *Quality Review—A Journal of the USP Practitioners Reporting Network,* by 1995 almost all pharmacies in the United States used computers to process prescriptions. Although the use of computers makes filling prescriptions faster and easier, and streamlines record keeping, computers have also been the source of some errors. The errors can be caused by incorrect data entry, an incorrect choice from a computer list, or software error. Incorrect entry of a prescription or an incorrect choice from a list of medications are human errors that can happen whether or not computers are used. However, some errors stem directly from software. In one case the programmer had used the same abbreviation (DOX100) to designate two different drugs. The incorrect medication lengthened one patient's hospital stay. Another program automatically printed "teaspoonful" when a liquid medication dose did not have a measure entered. This led to an infant being given an overdose of albuterol syrup. Other errors have occurred when software interpreted 1–2 (one to two) as one-half.

However, errors in software can be corrected. Generally, all drug errors decline when computers are introduced. Recently a study was done comparing drug errors before and after the introduction of a computerized prescription entry system in a large hospital. The study looked at errors in drug ordering, administration, and dispensing. Simply introducing a computerized order system cut errors at all three stages. Total errors fell 55 percent. Errors in transcription fell 84 percent. Another study compared adverse drug events in a 726-bed hospital before and after the introduction of computerized drug ordering. It found 126 errors in the first phase of the study, which had not been caught, and caught 134 errors in the second phase of the study. From the first to the second phase of the study, transcription errors fell to five (84 percent) (Study: Computers cut mistakes in doctors' prescriptions, 1998). The reduction in errors is partly due to making orders legible. Second, the computer checks dosage to make sure it is appropriate. It also checks for each patient's drug allergies and any possible drug interactions.

Computer warning systems can be used to prevent adverse drug events (ADEs). Serious ADEs occur in about 7 percent of patients admitted to hospitals. Many of these are caused by a physician prescribing either the wrong drug or the wrong dosage, because of lack of knowledge of either the patient or the drug. In 1994, a computerized warning system was designed and put into place in one hospital. The hospital already had in place a database with patient information; the existing system warned of a patient's specific drug allergy and of adverse drug interactions. The new alert system added warnings of other likely ADEs. The warnings were printed out for the pharmacist, who could alert the prescribing physician if he or she believed it was necessary. Physicians reported that the computer-generated alerts made them aware of the potential danger in 44 percent of alerts.

According to the 1999 government report, "To Err Is Human," between 44,000 and 98,000 people die in U.S. hospitals each year as a result of medical errors. Seven thousand people die from medication errors both in and out of the hospital. Among the changes the report recommends to reduce medication errors is to "require that all hospitals and health care organizations *implement proven safety practices, such as the use of automated drug ordering systems*" (emphasis added) (Richardson, 1999). Four years after the release of the report, one of its authors states, "We've seen pockets of dramatic improvement. Some of the hospitals . . . have had 10-fold reductions in adverse drug events. But overall, we're a long way from the goal" ("Preventing Medical Errors," 2003). In 2003, one doctor estimated that 16% of physicians scribble illegible prescriptions (Darves, 2003). The Florida legislature even passed a bill in the spring of 2003 ordering doctors to improve their handwriting (Dorschner, 2003).

A Harvard-led study conducted in 2002 and 2003 surveyed several hundred patients in each of the following countries: the United States, Canada, the United Kingdom, Australia, and New Zealand. Twenty-five percent of the people reported that they had experienced either a medical mistake or an error in prescribing. The number of errors grows as the number of doctors seen rises (Dorschner, 2003). Several reports in 2003 stressed that the use of computers to write prescriptions and check for errors in dosage is crucial in reducing ADEs. Hand-held computers provide immediate access to drug databases and other information. They also make prescriptions legible.

The Automated Community Pharmacy

Although not yet in common use, fully automated pharmacy systems that can fill prescriptions do exist for community drug stores (Figures 8.1a–8.1f). Currently the use of these systems is expanding with the successful use of robotic systems in Veterans' Administration pharmacies and hospitals. A fully automated dispensing system involves the employment of a robot. In one such system, a prescription is entered into the pharmacy computer; the pharmacy computer, in turn, activates the pharmacy robot, which first determines what size vial is needed for the prescription from the

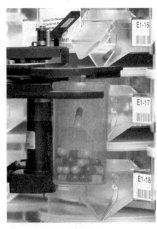

(a)

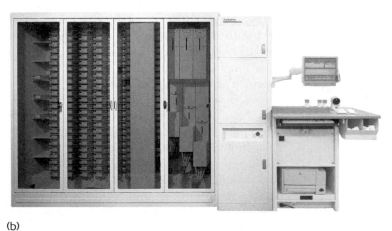

(b)

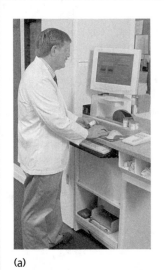

(c)

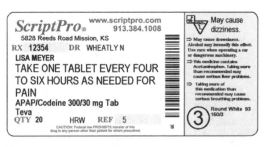

(d)

three available sizes. A robotic arm grips the correct size. One system has 200 cells, each containing a different drug. The arm is moved to the correct cell; the tablets or capsules are counted by a sensor and dropped into the vial. The computer prints a label and puts it on the vial, which is delivered via a conveyer belt to the pharmacist. The pharmacist uses a bar-code reader to scan the bar code on the label; an image of the medication and prescription information appears on the screen. The pharmacist puts the lid on and gives the customer the prescription. One robotic system can fill 150 prescriptions in an hour. Other robotic systems can fill prescriptions for liquid medications, as well as tablets and capsules.

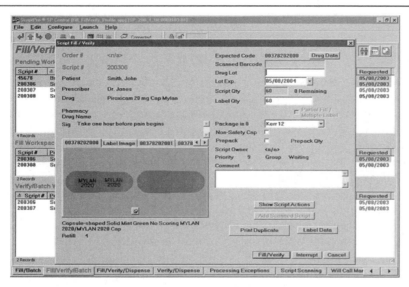

(e)

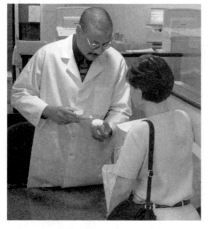

(f)

FIGURE 8.1 ScriptPro SP 200 Robotic Prescription Dispensing System. The ScriptPro fully automated prescription dispensing process begins by entering the prescription into the existing pharmacy computer system (a). Via the interface, the pharmacy computer sends the fill command to the SP 200 (b). The SP 200 robotic arm (c) then selects a standard vial from one of three vial dispensers in the system. The vial is automatically transported to the correct drug cell, the cell bar-code is scanned and the robotic arm engages the cell. The medication is dispensed and counted directly into the vial. The filled vial is automatically delivered to the ScriptPro print/apply labeling unit. At this point, the standard prescription information, a bar-code and USP auxiliary labels are printed and applied directly to the filled vial (d). The filled and labeled vial is then delivered on the conveyor to the pharmacist. The pharmacist scans the vial bar-code and verifies the prescription with an on-screen image of the medication and script information (e). The pharmacist then delivers the prescription to the patient, and completes the prescription filling process (f). Courtesy of ScriptPro.

Automating the Hospital Pharmacy

Hospitals are automating drug distribution systems. An automated hospital pharmacy presupposes the use of bar codes to identify drugs; it involves the use of robots in the hospital pharmacy to fill medication orders and/or the utilization of point-of-use dispensing units. A fully automated system may cost as much as $10 million, and take several years to install (Manning, 2002). Drugs are also being administered to patients by computerized infusion pumps. Automated dispensing systems can be centralized or decentralized. In a centralized system, robots are used in the hospital pharmacy to fill prescriptions. In a decentralized point-of-use dispensing system, drug cabinets, similar to ATM machines, are located throughout the hospital. Some hospitals use both robotics and automated point-of-use dispensing.

The Hospital Pharmacy Robot and Bar Codes

In a hospital pharmacy system using a pharmacy robot, medication orders are either faxed to the pharmacy and the information entered into the computer system or entered at a terminal connected with the pharmacy computer. The information includes the name of the patient, the medication, and the dose. Bar codes identify each dose of medication, and each dose is kept in a bag. (Any medication that is not identified by a bar code has to be dispensed by hand.) Each patient has a bin into which the robot drops his or her medication. If a bar code is unclear, the robot rejects the dose. The dosages are checked by technicians. In eight hours, one robot can do as much work as six or seven human technicians. The robot, its software, and five years of maintenance are extremely expensive. Hospital administrators maintain a robot still costs less than hiring six or seven human technicians for eight hours. Hospital managers, like managers in other businesses, see automation as a way to reduce costs, that is, staff, while maintaining service.

Each patient's medications are delivered to the nursing unit on a tray. As an added check on the accuracy of the computer, the bar codes on the patient's wristband and on the medication can be scanned. Dispensing errors are eliminated by using robots in the pharmacy. However, dispensing errors account for only 6 percent of medication errors. More than half occur at the prescribing stage and another third at the distribution stage.

The use of bar codes to identify medications and link them to patients also means that the robot is not only dispensing medication, but also keeping track of inventory. Additionally, it can automatically provide credit for medications, which are not used, and electronically order drugs when the supply is low.

Point-of-Use Drug Dispensing

Some computerized hospital pharmacies are using point-of-use dispensing of drugs—a decentralized automated system. A small computer attached to a large cabinet sits at the nursing unit. It is networked to the hospital pharmacy computer. A nurse types a password and the unit displays a list of patients; the nurse selects the patient and enters the drug order and the computer delivers it by opening the drawer containing the medication; the nurse then enters the name of the drug and closes the drawer. The computer keeps track of all drug transactions for billing and inventory purposes. It "counts, dispenses and tracks medications within the hospital." It can generate a variety of reports on patients, drug usage, and nurses. In 2003, the first automated drug dispensing units located in patients' rooms were introduced. Doctors can use them to enter prescriptions. The bedside system will scan the nurse's badge, the patient's wristband, and the medication's bar code. It is linked to databases of information that will help avoid medication errors. It can also keep track of inventory.

Point-of-use dispensing has several advantages over traditional manual dispensing. It shortens the time between the order for a medication and its delivery to the patient. One study found that the waiting time for a first dose of medication went from 45 minutes to one minute! Automating drug distribution improves patient care in other ways too. Drugs are more likely to be administered on schedule and significantly fewer doses are missed. Although apparently not reducing dispensing errors to zero like centralized robotic systems claim to do, one study found that a decentralized system decreased dispensing errors by almost one-third.

Decentralized computerized drug delivery has a positive financial impact for the hospital, making it more likely that patients are charged for the medications used. It also decreases the time nurses spend on medication-related activities, such as counting controlled substances, charting, documentation, and billing. A survey of nurses in a surgery unit that had introduced decentralized dispensing found that 80 percent wanted to keep the new system. It also decreased the time that pharmacists spend on problem resolution. Automation (although requiring an initial investment) can save a hospital as much as $1 million over five years in personnel time savings. About 100,000 hospitals are using this system nationwide ("Milestone Demonstrates Pyxis . . . ," 2002).

Point-of-use dispensing is also being introduced in clinics and doctors' offices. An automated drug-dispensing unit (something like a vending machine) contains approximately 90 percent of routinely prescribed drugs. A prescription can be entered by a doctor (with a password) and the medication automatically dispensed. However, there are states in which a doctor is not allowed to give a patient prescription drugs without a pharmacist.

TELEPHARMACY

Telepharmacy involves using a computer, a network connection, and a drug-dispensing unit to allow patients to obtain drugs outside of a traditional pharmacy, at, for example, a doctor's office or clinic. It should not be confused with the unregulated sale of prescriptions and drugs over the Internet. Telepharmacy links prescribing physicians with pharmacists via telecommunications lines. It may refer simply to the faxing of prescriptions from the prescribing doctor to the pharmacy for later pickup and the use of computers to check for adverse drug interactions. However, in a fully computerized telepharmacy system, the physician's and pharmacy's computers are directly linked, and the pharmacist remotely controls a drug cabinet at the physician's office. Once the pharmacist receives the prescription via a telecommunications link, a signal is sent to the remote drug cabinet to open a particular compartment. The dispensing cabinet (at the doctor's office) contains prepackaged drugs; each one is identified by a bar code. The software prints out a label and patient information and keeps track of inventory. A patient database includes the patient's age, allergies, drug use, diagnosis, and insurance provider. The software checks drug/drug interactions, drug/allergy interactions, and dosage, and it checks for duplicate prescriptions. Before the patient receives the medication, its bar code is scanned to make sure it is the right drug. The pharmacist and patient could then hold a video teleconsultation. Telepharmacy allows one pharmacist to serve a whole region.

There are several built-in safety checks. The bar code must be correct or the computer will not print a label, and, therefore, the patient will not get the drug. The computer also examines patient allergies, dangerous drug interactions, appropriate dosage, and expiration date; it immediately notifies the prescribing physician if there is a problem. The physician can, however, override the computer's warning. The cabinet in which the drugs are stored is secure and has alarms to guard against theft.

Although not yet in general use, telepharmacy promises to be especially helpful in rural areas and underserved urban neighborhoods where there is no accessible local pharmacy. Using a telepharmacy connection can mean that the patient walks out of the doctor's office with the medication in hand, having already teleconsulted with the pharmacist; neither patient nor pharmacist has to travel. It could prove to be particularly beneficial to populations who cannot travel easily. The elderly, for example, have a poor drug compliance record—due in part to their difficulty traveling. There are several other advantages to telepharmacy. A telepharmacy does not need to fill as many prescriptions as a conventional pharmacy to be cost effective. Entering prescriptions directly into a computer may cut down on dispensing errors caused by illegible handwriting. Handwritten signatures are no longer necessary. Since the July 2000 law making the digital signature equivalent to the handwritten signature, the doctor can prescribe without faxes and paper signatures. Dispensing drugs at the doctor's office guarantees that the prescription is filled. Pharmaceutical counseling ensures that the patient understands how to take the medication.

Today telepharmacy is slowly expanding (from less than half a dozen sites in 1998 to 100 in 2002) in part because of a shortage of pharmacists. The expansion is also due to government interest in telepharmacy as a cost-saving device, largely because of the use of generic medications, but also reflecting the higher efficiency of the pharmacist. The average price of a telepharmacy-filled prescription in Rockford, Iowa, is $19.93, compared with $30 at a pharmacy; the average price of antibiotics at a telepharmacy is $4 less than at a pharmacy; and the average price of an anti-inflammatory is $9.32, compared with $39.74 (Ukens, 1999). In 2002, the Department of Health and Human Services (HHS) funded a telepharmacy project designed to serve 13,500 low-income and rural patients. A pharmacist at the central location receives faxes of prescriptions and then sends a signal to a remote "vending machine" where a technician labels the bottle and gives it to the patient. There are five remote locations within a 100-mile radius (Ukens, 2002). The Veterans' Administration (VA), the US Department of Defense (DOD), and the Immigration and Naturalization Service (INS) are also testing telepharmacy systems (Page, 2000). The telepharmacy technology can link to the DOD's computerized medical system and automatically add prescriptions to a medical record.

There are problems with telepharmacy that could slow its expansion. Pharmacy has traditionally been subject to state regulation. Each state has different pharmacy regulations. The National Association of Boards of Pharmacy has model telepharmacy regulations, but only some states have adopted them.

DRUG DELIVERY ON A CHIP

Some medications can currently be delivered on an implanted chip. This is the focus of a great deal of research. The drug is embedded in a chip, which is surgically implanted in the patient. The drug may be released by diffusion. It may be embedded in a biodegradable material that releases as it degrades. One drug used to treat brain cancer is a biodegradable implant placed directly on the site from which the tumor was removed. The newest chip to be announced (October 2003) can deliver several medications. It can also deliver specific doses at predetermined times. The chip is in the early stages of development. Medications are embedded in polymers (plastics) that have already been approved by the FDA for other uses in humans. Thus far, the chips have been tested only on animals. Some of its potential uses include delivering an entire course of medication over a period of months, delivering a series of vaccines at the correct times, and delivering medication that needs to be taken continuously, including painkillers and medications for chronic conditions. This "pharmacy on a chip" is completely biodegradable. One advantage of using chips to deliver medication is that because they bypass the stomach, they avoid stomach upsets (Mitchell, 2003).

THE IMPACT OF INFORMATION TECHNOLOGY ON PHARMACY

Information technology is having a great impact on the field of pharmacy—affecting doctors, patients, pharmacists, and hospital management in different ways. The increasing use of computers requires doctors and pharmacists to be computer literate. The impact of automation on pharmacists is overwhelming. In both the hospital pharmacy and community drug store, robots can do what a human pharmacist has always done, that is, fill prescriptions. This allows pharmacists to be more involved in consulting with patients and physicians. In at least one hospital using a pharmacy robot, pharmacists now accompany doctors on rounds. However, hospitals using robots require fewer pharmacists; managers see this staff reduction as a benefit. It saves money, while maintaining services. It is unlikely that many pharmacists share this view.

The impact on patients appears to be beneficial. The Human Genome Project holds the promise of understanding the basis of diseases with a genetic link. This, combined with rational drug design may lead to the development of effective treatments and cures for many diseases. Automating drug dispensing in hospitals and drug stores has apparently reduced dispensing errors considerably.

Telepharmacy also affects patients, doctors, and pharmacists in different ways. Doctors can send a patient home with medication in hand, after teleconsulting with a pharmacist; patients do not need to travel long distances to fill prescriptions or consult with a pharmacist. Pharmacists can serve a much wider geographic area, and yet do not need to fill as many prescriptions to stay in business. Pharmacists need to achieve a high degree of computer literacy and familiarity with telecommunications and networks to be involved in telepharmacy.

SELECTED READING

Michelle Meadows. "Strategies to Reduce Medication Errors." *FDA Consumer* (May–June 2003).

IN THE NEWS

Strategies to Reduce Medication Errors

How the FDA Is Working to Improve Medication Safety and What You Can Do to Help

by Michelle Meadows

Since 1992, the Food and Drug Administration has received about 20,000 reports of medication errors. These are voluntary reports, so the number of medication errors that actually occur is thought to be much higher. There is no "typical" medication error, and health professionals, patients, and their families are all involved. Some examples:

A physician ordered a 260-milligram preparation of Taxol for a patient, but the pharmacist prepared 260 milligrams of Taxotere instead. Both are chemotherapy drugs used for different types of cancer and with different recommended doses. The patient died several days later, though the death couldn't be linked to the error because the patient was already severely ill.

An elderly patient with rheumatoid arthritis died after receiving an overdose of methotrexate—a 10-milligram daily dose of the drug rather than the intended 10-milligram weekly dose. Some dosing mix-ups have occurred because daily dosing of methotrexate is typically used to treat people with cancer, while low weekly doses of the drug have been prescribed for other conditions, such as arthritis, asthma, and inflammatory bowel disease.

One patient died because 20 units of insulin was abbreviated as "20 U," but the "U" was mistaken for a "zero." As a result, a dose of 200 units of insulin was accidentally injected.

A man died after his wife mistakenly applied six transdermal patches to his skin at one time. The multiple patches delivered an overdose of the narcotic pain medicine fentanyl through his skin.

A patient developed a fatal hemorrhage when given another patient's prescription for the blood thinner warfarin.

These and other medication errors reported to the FDA may stem from poor communication, misinterpreted handwriting, drug name confusion, lack of employee knowledge, and lack of patient understanding about a drug's directions. "But it's important to recognize that such errors are due to multiple factors in a complex medical system," says Paul Seligman, M.D., director of the FDA's Office of Pharmacoepidemiology and Statistical Science. "In most cases, medication errors can't be blamed on a single person."

Patient Safety Proposals

In March 2003, Health and Human Services Secretary Tommy G. Thompson announced two proposed rules from the FDA that will use state-of-the-art technology to improve patient safety. Here is a snapshot of each rule:

- **Bar codes:** Just as the technology is used in retail and other industries, required bar codes would contain unique identifying information about drugs. When used with bar code scanners and computerized patient information systems, bar code technology can prevent many medication errors, including administering the wrong drug or dose, or administering a drug to a patient with a known allergy.
- **Safety Reporting:** The proposed revamping of safety reporting requirements aims to enhance the FDA's ability to monitor and improve the safe use of drugs and biologics. The rule would improve the quality and consistency of safety reports, require the submission of all suspected serious reactions for blood and blood products, and require reports on important potential medication errors.

Computerized Physician Order Entry (CPOE)

Studies have shown that CPOE is effective in reducing medication errors. It involves entering medication orders directly into a computer system rather than on paper or verbally. The Institute for Safe Medication Practices conducted a survey of 1,500 hospitals in 2001 and found that about 3 percent of hospitals were using CPOE, and the number is rising. Eugene Wiener, M.D., medical director at the Children's Hospital of Pittsburgh, says, "There is no misinterpretation of handwriting, decimal points, or abbreviations. This puts everything in a digital world."

The Pittsburgh hospital unveiled its CPOE system in October 2002. Developed by the hospital and the Cemer Corporation in Kansas City, MO., Children'sNet has replaced most paper forms and prescription pads. Wiener says that, unlike with adults, most drug orders for children are generally based on weight. "The computer won't let you put an order in if the child's weight isn't in the system," he says, "and if the weight changes, the computer notices." The system also provides all kinds of information about potential drug complications that the doctor might not have thought about. "Doctors always have a choice in dealing with the alerts," Wiener says. "They can choose to move past an alert, but the alert makes them stop and think based on the specific patient indications."

CHAPTER SUMMARY

This chapter introduced the reader to the impact of information technology in the field of pharmacy.

- Computer technology is making a contribution to rational drug design. Because computers can do billions of calculations and then graphically represent the results, it is possible to create graphical models of a target molecule, for which a drug can be specifically designed.
- Bioinformatics is the application of information technology to biology.
- The Human Genome Project is leading to an understanding of the molecular bases of diseases that have a genetic link. This knowledge has led to the development of drugs that are currently in the testing stages.
- Drug trials can be simulated using computers, so that actual trials take less time and cost less, and are more likely to be successful.
- Information technology is changing the way pharmacies do business.
  - Computers are used in the corner drug store to provide information for customers and pharmacists. Some drug stores are fully computerized, with robots filling the prescriptions.
  - In hospitals two computerized pharmacy systems exist (and may coexist).
    - A centralized system uses robots in the hospital pharmacy to fill drug orders typed in on terminals. The drugs are identified by bar codes. Each patient's medications are then delivered to the unit.
    - In a decentralized point-of-use dispensing system, computers attached to cabinets sit in various places in the hospital. A nurse may enter a password and type in a medication order; the drawer with the medication opens and the nurse can remove it.
    - Both centralized and decentralized systems cut down on drug dispensing errors and on the amount of time personnel spend on medication-related activity.
  - Telepharmacy involves the linking of a pharmacist with a remote drug cabinet in a doctor's office via telecommunications lines.
- Information technology is affecting doctors, patients, pharmacists, and administrators in different ways.

KEY TERMS

antisense technology
bioinformatics
biotechnology
computer-assisted trial
design (CATD)

Food and Drug
Administration
(FDA)
Human Genome Project
Physiome Project

rational drug design
ribonucleic acid (RNA)
RNA interference (RNAi)
scientific visualization
telepharmacy

REVIEW QUESTIONS

Multiple Choice

1. The creation of medications using computers to create a model of the target molecule and design a medication to inhibit or stimulate its work is called _____.

   A. Biotechnology
   B. Rational drug design
   C. Visualization
   D. None of the above

2. The _____ is a project attempting to understand the genetic makeup of the human being.

   A. International Genome Project
   B. National Institute of Health Project
   C. Genetic Script
   D. Human Genome Project

3. A centralized computerized hospital pharmacy system involves the use of _____.

   A. Bar codes to identify drugs
   B. Robots
   C. A and B
   D. None of the above

4. Which of the following is true of decentralized point-of-use dispensing?

   A. It decreases the waiting time for the first dose of a drug.
   B. It increases the likelihood that drugs are administered on schedule.
   C. It decreases dispensing errors.
   D. All of the above

5. The linking of a drug cabinet in a doctor's office with a pharmacist via telecommunications lines is called _____.

   A. Telemedicine
   B. Telepharmacy
   C. Remote pharmacy
   D. Robotic pharmacy

6. Information technology has made the Human Genome Project possible by _____.

   A. Enabling scientists to keep track of genes as they are identified, and allowing findings to be immediately communicated via the Internet
   B. Making pharmacy robots available internationally
   C. Keeping track of new drugs as they enter clinical trials
   D. Keeping records of the results of clinical drug trials

7. Telepharmacy raises certain legal problems associated with _____.
    A. The prescribing of drugs that are not FDA approved
    B. Interstate licensing of pharmacists
    C. A doctor prescribing medications
    D. None of the above
8. The Human Genome Project may lead to _____.
    A. A more complete understanding of genetics
    B. More accurate predictions of who is likely to develop a disease with a genetic basis
    C. Both A and B
    D. None of the above
9. The use of computers to simulate drug trials _____.
    A. Means that we do not need actual clinical trials
    B. Means actual clinical trials are more likely to succeed
    C. Helps save both time and money
    D. B and C
10. DNA provides a blueprint of genetic information. _____ helps create the proteins.
    A. Biotechnology
    B. RNA
    C. TNA
    D. None of the above

True/False Questions

1. Errors in software can lead to errors in filling prescriptions. _____
2. Understanding the genetic basis of a disease can lead to the development of an effective drug. _____
3. Hospital pharmacy robots can dispense *any* drug with a bar code. _____
4. Decentralized hospital dispensing units reduce dispensing errors to zero. _____
5. Telepharmacy allows one pharmacist to serve a large geographic area. _____
6. Automation of pharmacy may lead to unemployment among pharmacists. _____
7. Antisense technology attempts to treat cancer by turning off a gene that keeps cells alive. _____
8. Biotechnology sees the human body as a collection of molecules. _____
9. Computers have helped in the development of drugs used to treat AIDS. _____
10. Computer-assisted trial design means that real clinical trials are not needed. _____

Critical Thinking

1. Discuss the advantages and disadvantages of the introduction of computers in a local pharmacy,
    a. from the pharmacist's point-of-view, and
    b. from the customer's point-of-view

2. As the administrator of a small hospital, discuss the advantages and disadvantages of introducing a centralized computerized hospital pharmacy system using robots.
3. Telepharmacy could prove to be a benefit to elderly patients who have difficulty traveling. However, privacy, security, and legal issues may have to be settled before telepharmacy becomes an established part of health care. Discuss this statement. Consider licensing issues and the lack of security of networked communications in your answer.

SOURCES

"Automated Pharmacy Reduces Cost and Eliminates Errors." http://www.tech80.com/applications/ah.html (1996–1999; June 9, 1999).

Baase, Sara. *A Gift of Fire.* Upper Saddle River, NJ: Prentice-Hall, pp. 22–23.

Barker, Kenneth N., Bill G. Felkey, Elizabeth A. Flynn, and Jim L. Carper. "White Paper on Automation in Pharmacy." http://www.ascp.com (March 1998; October 24, 2003).

Borel, Jacques, and Karen L. Rascati. "Effect of an Automated, Nursing Unit-Based Drug-Dispensing Device on Medication Errors." American Society of Health System Pharmacists, Inc. Originally published in the *American Journal of Health System Pharmacy* 52 (September 1, 1995): 1875–79; Article Review and Commentary (September 1, 1995; October 24, 2003).

"Cardinal Health Installs New Point-of-Care Technology System in Huron Valley-Sinai Hospital." pyxis.com (March 6, 2003; August 28, 2003).

"Cardinal Health Introduces Health Care's First Patient Room Automated Dispensing System for Medications and Supplies." pyxis.com (June 2, 2003; August 28, 2003).

Cefalu, William T. and William Weir. "New Technologies in Diabetes Care." patientcareonline.com (September 2003; October 24, 2003).

"Center to Offer Quick, Reliable Source for Genetic Information." National Genome Research Institute. genome.gov (n.d.; August 17, 2003).

Chervokas, Jason, and Tom Watson. "Doctors Build a Community Online." *CyberTimes,* February 6, 1998. http://www.nytimes.com/library/cyber/nation/020698nation.html (February 6, 1998; July 16, 1998).

Clark, Chapin. "Fedco Unit Pharmacy Going Robotic." *Supermarket News,* (February 2, 1998).

"Computer-Assisted Trial Design." http://www.Pharsight.com/html/services/srv.catd.php (2003; October 24, 2003).

"Computerized Order Entry System Reduces Serious Medication Errors by 50 Percent: Using Computers Can Lower Costs and Improve Quality." Science News Update, October 21, 1998. http://www.ama-assn.org/sci-pubs/sci-news/1998/snr1021.htm#joc80319 (October 21, 1998; October 24, 2003).

"Computers: Errors In—Errors Out." *Quality Review* 48 (August 1995). http://www.usp.org (August 1995; October 24, 2003).

Darves, Bonnie. "Seven Simple Steps to Prevent Outpatient Drug Errors." American College of Physicians *Observer.* acponline.org (June 2003; October 28, 2003).

Dorschner, John. "Study Finds Healthcare Error Prone." http://www.miami.com/mld/miamiherald/5793072.htm (May 6, 2003; October 29, 2003).

"FDA Approves Herceptin for Breast Cancer," http://www.pslgroup.com/dg/b1c82.htm (September 29, 1998; October 24, 2003).

"FDA Approves Xolair, Biotechnology Breakthrough for Asthma." gene.com (June 20, 2003; September 1, 2003).

Fleiger, Ken. "Getting SMART: Drug Review in the Computer Age." *FDA Consumer.* http://www.fda.gov/fdac/features/895_smart.html (October 1995; October 24, 2003).

Fletcher, Amy. "Hospital Drug Delivery Systems Take High-Tech Route." http://denver.bizjournals.com (August 8, 2003; October 29, 2003).

"From Maps to Medicine: About the Human Genome Research Project." http://www.nhgri.nih.gov/Policy_and_public_affairs/Communications/Publications/Maps_to_medicine/about.html (August 9, 2000; October 24, 2003).

"Genentech Presents Positive Preliminary Six-Month Data from Phase Ib/II Study for Lucentis in Age-Related Macular Degeneration (AMD)." gene.com (August 18, 2003; September 1, 2003).

"Genentech Receives FDA Fast-Track Designation for Avastin." gene.com (June 26, 2003; September 1, 2003).

Gump, Michael D. "Robot Technology Improves VA Pharmacies—U.S. Medicine Interviews." usmedicine.com (July 2001; September 25, 2002).

"Health Plans for Virtual Human." BBC News. news.bbc.co.uk (May 17, 1999; September 1, 2003).

Human Genome Resources. NCBI.com (2003; August 17, 2003).

"Information Technology Is One Key to Improving Patient Safety." ahcpr.gov/research/Sept03/0903RA19.htm (September 2003; October 28, 2003).

Jehlen, Alan. "Preventing Medical Errors." *American Teacher.* aft.org (May/June 2003; October 28, 2003).

Karash, Julius A. "Robots Fit the Prescription." *Kansas City Star,* January 14, 1998, p. B3.

Manning, Margie. "Computers to Replace Docs' Scribbles at Barnes-Jewish: $10 Million System Will Place Orders for Drugs, Tests; Should Be in Place within Three Years." stlouis.bizjournals.com (March 4, 2002; October 29, 2003).

Marietti, Charlene. "Robots Hooked on Drugs: Robotic Automation Expands Pharmacy Services, 11/97." *Healthcare Informatics.* http://www.healthcare-informatce.com/issues/1997/11_97/robots.htm (November 1997; October 24, 2003).

"Milestone Demonstrates Pyxis Corporation's Leadership in Development of Automated Medication Technology for Patient Safety." pyxis.com (January 10, 2002; August 28, 2003).

Mitchell, Steve. "Scientists Create 'Pharmacy in a Chip.'" http://www.nlm.nih.gov/medlineplus (October 19, 2003; October 26, 2003).

Neergaard, Lauran. "DNA to Aid in Tailoring Prescription for Patient." *Star-Ledger,* November 3, 2003, p. 23.

Ouellette, Jennifer, "Biomaterials Facilitate Medical Breakthroughs." American Institute of Physics. www.aip.org (October/November 2001; October 24, 2003).

Page, Douglas. "Drug Topics." addsinc.com (March 20, 2000; August 18, 2003).

"Physicians Hospital of El Paso Set to Deploy Pyxis Safetynet Technology to Reduce Medical Errors." pyxis.com (October 10, 2002; August 28, 2003).

Pollack, Andrew. "Drug Testers Turn to 'Virtual Patients' as Guinea Pigs." *New York Times,* November 10, 1998, pp. F1, F10.

———. "Merck and Partner Form Alliance to Develop Drugs Based on RNA." nyt.com (September 9, 2003; September 10, 2003).

———. "Mixed Data Leave Doubts on Cancer Drug." nyt.com (September 12, 2003; September 12, 2003).

Powell, Jennifer Heldt. "Long-Distance Remedy: ADDS System Indispensible." *Boston Herald.* addsinc.com (June 14, 1999; August 18, 2003).

"Preventing Death and Injury from Medical Errors Requires Dramatic, System-Wide Changes." National Academies. news@nas.edu (November 29, 1999; August 27, 2003).

"Preventing Medical Errors." *On Campus.* www.aft.org (May–June 2003; May 14, 2004).

Raschke, R. A., B. Gollihare, T. A. Wunderlich, J. R. Guidry, A. I. Leibowitz, J. C. Pierce, L. Lemelson, M. A. Heisler, and C. Susong. "A Computer Alert System to Prevent Injury from Adverse Drug Events." *JAMA* (October 21, 1998): 1317–20.

Reducing and Preventing Adverse Drug Events To Decrease Hospital Costs. Research in Action, Issue 1. AHRQ Publication Number 01-0020, March 2001. Agency for Healthcare Research and Quality, Rockville, MD. http://www.ahrq.gov/qual/aderia/aderia.htm (March 2001; June 28, 2004).

Richardson, William C. "To Err Is Human: Building a Safer Health System." news@nas.edu (December 1, 1999; August 28, 2003).

"RNA Structure Database, The." RNABase.org (September 10, 2003; September 11, 2003).

"Rx for Speedy Service." http://www.addsinc.com/news/media/insidetrack-rxspeed.html (September 20, 1997; October 12, 2003).

Sardinha, Carol. "Electronic Prescribing: The Next Revolution in Pharmacy." *Journal of Managed Care Pharmacy,* http://www.amcp.org/jmcp/vol4/num1/spotlight.html (January–February 1998; October 24, 2003).

Schwarz, Harold, and Bret Brodowy. "Implementation and Evaluation of an Automated Dispensing System" (Abstract). *American Journal of Health-System Pharmacy* 52 (April 15, 1995): 823–28. ncbi.nlm.nih.gov (1998; October 24, 2003).

"Significant Milestones in Biotechnology." Genentech Inc. http://www.gene.com (2000; October 24, 2003).

Sipkoff, Martin, "Telepharmacy Helps Improve Efficiency." qualityindicator.com (February 2001; March 13, 2003).

"Spokane Pharmacists Test Rx Vending Machine Dispensing." addsinc.com (February 2002; August 18, 2003).

Stephenson, Joan. "Targeting Medical Errors." American Medical Association 283, no. 3. abs.ca (January 19, 2000; October 12, 2003).

"Study: Computers Cut Mistakes in Doctors' Prescriptions." CNN.com (October 20, 1998; October 12, 2003).

"Tarceva (erlotnib HCl) Phase II Clinical Trials Initiated in Patients with Malignant Glioma." gene.com (August 8, 2003; September 1, 2003).

"Thompson Approves Demos to Expand Safety-Net Patients' Access to Prescription Drugs and Pharmacy Services, Lower Drug Prices," HHS News, U.S. Department of Health and Human Services. addsinc.com (December 18, 2001; August 18, 2003).

Ukens, Carol. "Dispensing by Remote Control Cuts Drug Costs." addsinc.com (July 5, 1999; August 18, 2003).

———. "Eckerd Uses Technology to Help Provide Pharmacist Care." *Drug Topics,* June 1, 1998, p. 76.

———. "Pharmacy Shortage Boosts Telepharmacy." addsinc.com (June 3, 2002; August 18, 2003).

Wade, Nicholas. "Scientists Discover First Gene Tied to Stroke." nyt.com (September 22, 2003; September 22, 2003).

"What Is a Helix? And What Is RNA and DNA . . ." http://www.chemistry-school.info (n.d.; September 10, 2003).

"What Is RNA?" strategis.ic.gc.ca (October 16, 2000; September 10, 2003).

Zdrakas, Chris. "Robot Gives Customer Service New Meaning." afmc.wpafb.af.mil (August 6, 2002; September 25, 2002).

CHAPTER 9

Computerized Medical Devices, Assistive Technology, and Prosthetic Devices

OUTLINE

- **Learning Objectives**
- **Overview**
- **Computerized Medical Instruments**
  - *Computerized Devices in Optometry/Ophthalmology*
- **Assistive Devices**
- **Augmentative Communications Devices**
  - *Environmental Control Systems*
- **Prosthetic Devices**
- **CFES Technology**
- **Risks Posed by Implants**
- **Conclusion**
- **Selected Readings**
- **Chapter Summary**
- **Key Terms**
- **Review Questions**
  - *Multiple Choice*
  - *True/False Questions*
  - *Critical Thinking*
- **Sources**

LEARNING OBJECTIVES

Upon completion of this chapter, you will be able to

- Describe the contribution made to the design of medical devices by information technology and be able to discuss the advantages of computerized medical monitoring systems over their predecessors.
- Describe the use of computerized devices in delivering medications.

- Discuss the Americans with Disabilities Act of 1990 and be able to discuss the impact digital technology has had on assistive devices for people with physical challenges.
  - List assistive devices for those with impaired vision, speech, hearing, and mobility.
  - Discuss speech recognition devices, speech synthesizers, and screen readers.
- Describe the contributions computer technology has made to the development of prosthetics.
  - Discuss the contributions of computer technology to the improvement of myo-electric limbs.
  - Discuss the contributions computer technology has made to improving sight for the blind and hearing for the deaf.
- Define functional electrical stimulation.
  - List its uses in implanted devices such as pacemakers.
  - Discuss its use in simulating physical workouts for paralyzed muscles and restoring movement to paralyzed limbs.
- Discuss the risks posed by implants.

OVERVIEW

Digital technology, particularly the microprocessor, has had an enormous impact on the creation, design, and manufacture of medical devices, adaptive devices, and prosthetics. Computers have improved the design of some devices with health care applications and made possible a whole range of new ones. In hospitals and medical offices, computerized medical instruments with embedded microprocessors are more accurate than their predecessors. In the workplace and the home, the impact of information technology on people who are physically challenged is tremendous. **Assistive,** or **adaptive, technology** allows some people with disabilities to work and/or live independently.

Prosthetic devices (replacement limbs and organs) that contain motors and respond to electrical signals existed prior to computers. However, prosthetic devices designed and manufactured with the help of computers and containing microprocessors are more sensitive, lighter, and more flexible and can work almost as well as natural limbs. **Computerized functional electrical stimulation (CFES or FES)** is technology that involves delivering low-level electrical stimulation to muscles. Used for many years in pacemakers, CFES is now being used to strengthen muscles paralyzed by spinal cord injury or stroke. CFES is being used experimentally to restore the ability to stand and walk to paraplegics.

COMPUTERIZED MEDICAL INSTRUMENTS

Computerized medical instruments are "electronic devices equipped with microprocessors [which] provide direct patient services such as monitoring . . . [and] administering medication or treatment" (Kreig, 2001). Computerized drug delivery systems are used to give medications. Insulin pumps include a battery operated pump and a computer chip. The pump is not automatic. However, the chip allows the user to control the amount of insulin administered. Insulin is administered via a plastic tube inserted under the skin; the tube is changed every two or three days. The pump is worn externally and continually delivers insulin according to the user's program. In March 2001, the FDA approved a new device for glucose testing. It is worn like a watch and takes fluid through the skin using electric currents; electrodes measure the glucose. The measurements are taken every 20 minutes, and an alarm goes off if the levels are too low. Tests showed that this method was not as accurate as the finger prick, and is not meant to replace it, but to reveal trends. Electronic IV units not only are programmable, but also can detect incorrect flow and sound an alarm. Some units can be programmed to administer several drugs through several channels. Intravenous anesthesia can be administered via a mechanical syringe infusion pump, controlled by complex and sophisticated software.

Computerized monitoring systems that collect data directly from patients via sensors have been used for many years. These devices can provide continuous oversight of a patient's condition and can be programmed to sound an alarm under certain conditions to notify human personnel of a change. Computerized **physiological monitoring systems** that analyze blood, **arrhythmia monitors** that monitor heart rates, **pulmonary monitors** that measure blood flow through the heart and respiratory rate, **fetal monitors** that measure the heart rate of the fetus, and **neonatal monitors** that monitor infant heart and breathing rates are devices that are standard and accepted.

Computerized instruments are both more accurate and more reliable than their predecessors. For example, an infusion pump can be set at the desired rate and that rate will be maintained. Its predecessor, whose flow had to be estimated, could have its rate changed by the patient's movements. Computerized cardiac monitors are able, unlike their predecessors, to distinguish between cardiac arrest and a wire coming loose.

Monitoring devices may or may not be linked to a network. Stand-alone devices include IV pumps, EKG and cardiac monitors, defibrillators, and TPR and blood pressure monitors. When devices are networked, patients can be monitored from a central location within the hospital such as a nurses' station, or even from a physician's home. Networked devices can interact with each other; for example, a cardiac monitor can communicate with a medication delivery device. Networked equipment is most common in emergency rooms, operating rooms, and critical and intensive care units. Since a network makes patient information immediately available anywhere in the hospital and allows a specialist to consult with the emergency room online, it can reduce response time in emergencies.

Computerized Devices in Optometry/Ophthalmology

An ophthalmologist is a doctor who treats eye diseases. An optometrist examines the eye and prescribes glasses. Computerized devices help make eye care, from preliminary vision testing to surgery, more precise. Computerized instruments are used to measure refractive error and the shape of the cornea. The **Optomap Panoramic200** can examine the retina without dilation, using low-powered red and green lasers. The image can be reviewed right away and is larger than that produced by conventional examination. It can help in the early detection of retinal tears, macular degeneration, and diabetic retinopathy. Tools called **biomicroscopes** are used for diagnosis of cataracts. **Tonometers** measure eye pressure. **Corneal topography** uses a computer to create an accurate three-dimensional map of the cornea, so the health care professional can see the shape and power of the cornea. The **Heidelberg Retinal Tomograph (HRT)** uses lasers to scan the retina, resulting in a three-dimensional description. This technique can detect glaucoma before any loss of vision. **GDx Access** uses an infrared laser to measure the thickness of the retinal nerve fiber. It is used for the early detection of glaucoma. Computers help to make cataract surgery more precise. In such surgery, the eye's lens is replaced by an intra-ocular lens (IOL). The most precise measurements are needed to determine which IOL to implant. **Optical biometry** refers to the IOL calculations. Traditionally ultrasound was used for the measurement; it required anesthesia. The IOLmaster takes precise measures in a shorter time and requires no anesthesia. The **Tracey Visual Function Analyzer** measures how well you can see by measuring how your eye focuses light. This data helps in surgical or laser vision correction. Computers are also used to custom design contact lenses.

ASSISTIVE DEVICES

The **Americans with Disabilities Act of 1990** prohibits discrimination against people with disabilities and requires that businesses with more than 15 employees provide "reasonable accommodation" to allow the disabled to perform their jobs. Thus, employers are required to provide not only entrance ramps for people in wheelchairs, but also hardware and software that make computers usable by people with disabilities. Many assistive devices have been developed. Adaptive technology makes it possible for people with disabilities to exercise control over their home and work environments. Some assistive devices allow people with physical challenges to work with computers and other office equipment. Others simply improve the quality of life. For example, at Boston University, scientists are developing a system based on computer-generated noise that helps elderly people keep their balance. It sends random vibrations to the feet, which automatically adjust their balance.

Wheelchairs are being developed that not only help move people around, but also climb stairs and allow them to reach a high shelf. The iBOT wheelchair stands up on its back wheels if the user needs to climb stairs, and raises the seat to allow reaching. An even smarter wheelchair is being developed. It includes sensors and a computer, and the user can simply tell it where to go or use a touch panel. The wheelchair finds its way, using laser radar to find objects in its path; a computer calculates a new path if necessary.

Computer technology can help those with impaired vision, hearing, speech, and mobility. People with low or no vision can use speech recognition systems as input and speech synthesizers for output. Brain input systems are being developed for people who lack the muscle control to use alternative input devices.

Assistive technology encompasses many areas. People with low vision can use a large type display on a monitor. Braille keyboards allow the blind to type. Blind users can use keyboard alternatives to mouse clicks as commands (e.g., [ALT]-F-O, instead of clicking on the open icon). In 2003, a Braille phone organizer was developed. It combines the functions of the cell phone, note taker, and wireless Internet connector. It can receive information and either read it to the user or allow the user to read it in Braille. Text can be entered using its Braille keyboard.

Speech recognition is useful for people who do not have the use of their hands and for the vision impaired. It promises that you can give computer commands or dictate text. Speech recognition hardware includes a microphone and a chip inside the computer that converts the spoken word to digital data that the computer can process. The digitized word is compared with a database of words in the computer's memory; if a match is found, the word is recognized. Speech recognition systems enable the user to give voice commands to their computers instead of clicking with a mouse, and to write, edit, and format text documents by dictating instead of typing. Although great progress has been made in recent years, speech recognition is not perfect, particularly with continuous speech. **Discrete speech recognition systems** require the user to pause between words. Although they allow more natural speech, **continuous speech recognition systems** require more powerful computers. Recently, a great deal of progress has been made, and error rates have dropped to less than 1 percent. The software still has problems recognizing lower voices, some accents, and can be confused by incorrect grammar and background noise. The most perfect speech recognition system would still not be able to distinguish between some English words and phrases. "Hyphenate" sounds exactly like "–8" (hyphen 8); "the right or left" sounds like "the writer left." However, these errors can now be corrected with speech commands. In an attempt to improve speech recognition, scientists at IBM are trying to teach computers to lip-read. Using cameras, the computer would "see" the speaker, and ideally be able to use facial clues just as human beings do. A computer program would analyze the speech using both audio and visual clues.

Speech recognition systems can be **speaker-independent** or **speaker-dependent**. A speaker-independent system recognizes a limited number of commands spoken in standard North American English. A speaker-dependent system needs to be trained to recognize the user's speech patterns. Some systems have large vocabularies (over 100,000 words) and can be used to create, edit, and format text documents, as well as to control the computer with spoken commands. Other programs serve a specific function. There are programs, which allow the user to surf the net by saying the name of a page with a hypertext link or telling the program to go forward or back, up or down, home, and so on. With some, you can dictate characters one-by-one, allowing the entry of a URL.

Using **page scanners, speech synthesizers**, and **screen reader software**, printed text can be digitized and input and then read aloud by the computer. A scanner converts printed text into a form the computer can accept as input, that is, it digitizes it. Speech synthesis refers to the ability of a computer to talk; voice output devices turn digital data into speechlike sounds, allowing the computer to talk or read *to* a vision-impaired user or speak *for* a speech-impaired user. Speech synthesis requires both hardware and software. The speech synthesizer is really a computer in itself with a processor, memory, and an output device. The software is loaded into the synthesizer's memory, and the microprocessor generates speech output. It translates binary code to speech. A speaker and amplifier are also necessary. Screen reader software tells the speech synthesizer what to say, for example, to read the text description of an icon.

People with impaired vision are not the only users of speech recognition software. People who have lost the use of their hands also find it useful; instead of typing, they can talk to the computer. However, it is especially difficult to control a mouse with voice commands. DragonDictate uses a numbered grid on the screen. The user can pick a section and the mouse moves to it; the section is subdivided further and the user can pick a section again. This process continues until the mouse is where the user wants it. Other input devices include the **head mouse**, which moves the cursor according to the user's head motions. **Puff straws** allow people to control the mouse with their mouths. Some computers allow input through eye movement. The newest eye input system does not require the user to stare at letter after letter, but allows the eye to move down a column of letters and stop on one. The chosen letter floats on the screen and the software predicts the next most likely letters. For example, if the user selected a q, u would be the next most likely letter. After the u, the next letter would be an a, e, i, or o. Users of this system can type at 25 words per minute, compared with 15 wpm using an onscreen keyboard. Perhaps most amazing are programs that attempt to translate electrical impulses from the brain into a mouse click. A quadriplegic can, after a period of training, click a mouse by contracting facial muscles or simply thinking. In 2003, a system that enabled a user to give a command by furrowing his or her brow on which a sensor was taped was demonstrated. Robotic arms and computer mice could be controlled using the sensor. Paralyzed stroke patients could speak on the phone.

Hearing impairment is not a barrier to computer use. However, computers do expand the means of communication that hearing-impaired people can access. Computers can be used as text telephones and can send and receive e-mail. Special modems can communicate with both **text telephones** and computers. Computer-aided transcription makes use of a typist entering verbal communications at a meeting. The communications are then displayed as text on a monitor.

AUGMENTATIVE COMMUNICATIONS DEVICES

An **augmentative communication device** is any device that helps a person communicate. Medicare began covering these devices in 2002. Those who lack the ability to speak or whose speech is impaired can have a computer speak for them. The device should allow the user to communicate basic needs, carry on conversations, work with a computer, and complete assignments for work or school. It should work with environmental controls at home and also travel with the user. It should enable the user to communicate with anyone, and say anything. It should be easy to use. There are devices that allow the user to type a message on a traditional keyboard and the computer speaks aloud. Some keyboards can be easily operated by one finger. Other devices, as you recall, allow the user to select letters by gazing at an area on the screen that displays the characters. For people whose speech is impaired, there are devices that enhance speech—making the unintelligible comprehensible—and allow normal communication. Many of these devices are user-friendly, that is, easy for people with no computer background to use. Some are specifically designed for children, allowing the user to move an electric pointer to select a picture symbol. Some devices for children have the words organized by part of speech, the English word appearing above the symbol. These devices include synthesized voices. More sophisticated devices included spelling, word prediction, and preprogrammed messages. Portable devices allow the user to communicate anywhere. A device, which the user wears on a belt, allows a user to communicate by pressing buttons to play prerecorded messages and carry on simple conversations.

Work is being done to develop brainwave control of alternative communication. Many people suffer from conditions that result in uncontrollable muscle activity. All alternative interfaces, including head and eye-tracking, chin switches, puff straws, and voice activation, depend on the user's muscle control. However, if the user lacks muscle control, devices are being tried that magnify brainwaves and allow the user to use brainwaves to control a cursor! The neural implant transmits brain waves over wires to an amplifier outside the brain. Chips have been surgically implanted in the brains of locked-in stroke patients, allowing them to communicate. Some researchers predict that brainwave input with sensors attached to the forehead (not implanted) will be a viable method to use in the future (Junker, 2003).

Environmental Control Systems

Environmental control systems help physically challenged people control their environments. Speech recognition technology can be used in the home to control appliances. Butler-in-a-Box has been made by Mastervoice since 1986. It not only understands and obeys voice commands, but also responds in a human voice. Using this system one can control home appliances with voice commands. It also acts as a speaker phone which will dial or answer calls on command. Other environmental control systems allow the installation of a single switch to control the operation of several appliances (including other controllers). A device even exists that holds the book the user is reading and turns the pages.

Environmental control systems can be used to control any electrical appliance in the home. This would include lights, telephones, computers, appliances, infrared devices, security systems, sprinklers, doors, curtains, and electric beds. Voice, joysticks, or switches may control the system. This may enable physically challenged people to live independently at home. One small study reported that 27 out of the 29 people with spinal injuries who used an ECS for one year "reported that it increased their independence" (Smith, 1999, pp. 7–9). Other studies found similar results. Several phones have been developed. It should be noted that all these systems required that the user be trained and comfortable with the technology and that the technology be reliable.

Another newer use of environmental controls is to help in language development in children. Many environmental controls include infrared capability. One possibility is using an action toy that moves back and forth to teach the concepts of backward and forward or fast/slow. In toys that require children to take turns, words such as My turn/Your turn could be taught (Anderson, 2003). Research is also being done into the possibility of using augmentative communication devices for patients who are only voiceless for a short time, due to illness or surgery.

PROSTHETIC DEVICES

Prostheses are devices that attempt to replace natural body parts or organs. **Myoelectric** limbs—artificial limbs containing motors and responding to the electrical signals transmitted by the residual limb to electrodes mounted in the socket—predate computers. However, computer-related research has improved myoelectric limbs and had an immense impact on prosthetics in general. Developments related to computers include the tiny circuitry used by the sensors that receive the electrical signals and the motors that move the limb, the use of computers in the design and manufacture of limbs, and the improvement of the sensors used in prostheses.

Today, microprocessors can be embedded in a prosthetic limb and make the limb more useful and flexible. Sensors are attached to muscles in the residual limb. The patient must be able to control these muscles. Contracting the muscles generates electrical impulses. A microprocessor processes and amplifies the electrical impulses, sending them as control signals to the prosthesis. The microprocessor controls the tiny motor that moves the artificial limb. Combined with natural-looking prostheses, the results can be a lifelike limb.

Computer-aided design and manufacturing (CAD/CAM) systems also improve prostheses by making the fit better. The artificial limb must be fitted to the natural limb. CAD/CAM systems have been developed to design both the socket and limb. With CAD/CAM, thousands of measurements can be taken and a three-dimensional model created on the computer screen to create a perfect custom fit for each patient (Figure 9.1). CAD/CAM is also used in dentistry to help create individually fitted prostheses.

Computers have made other advances possible. A knee socket has been developed which includes a computer chip that allows patients to walk naturally. Energy-storing feet contain plastic springs or carbon fibers, which are designed to help move the prosthesis. A relatively new lower leg prosthesis is called the C-leg or computerized leg. It includes a prosthetic knee and shin system controlled by a microprocessor. It is made of lightweight carbon fiber and gets its power from a rechargeable battery. With a traditional prosthesis, the user has to think about each step. But the C-leg analyzes gait 50 times per second; it anticipates movement, and thus thinks for the patient. It is supposed to adjust to uneven ground by itself, but

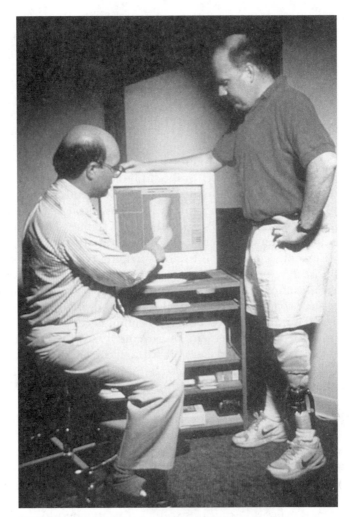

FIGURE 9.1   The CAPOD system allows the use of computer
technology to custom design prostheses.
Courtesy of Solaris Health Systems

results from studies are mixed. It requires less energy for walking at speeds slower
or faster than usual, but not at the walker's usual speed. The user does not have to
think about changing walking speed. In small studies, patient satisfaction is found
to be high. Most study participants chose to keep the C-leg as opposed to a conventional prosthesis.

    People with computerized prosthetic limbs not only walk but also can play
sports, run, climb mountains, and—using a prosthetic hand developed at Rutgers

University in 1998 with fingers that can be controlled separately—even play the piano! Soon prosthetic limbs will include sensors that allow a person to feel hot and cold. Temperature sensors in the prosthesis would send signals to electrodes on the natural limb. The information is sent to the brain, which registers sensation. Sense-of-feel systems are also being developed so that breakable objects can be manipulated.

The FDA has approved the testing of retinal implants. In a healthy eye, the retina changes light into electrical signals. The retinal implant contains thousands of light detectors and will also change light into electric signals. Currently scientists around the world are studying computer chips that will replace the retina. One major disagreement is where the chip should be implanted: under the retina close to light-detecting cells or near the retinal layer which sends nerve impulses to the brain. The way light is sent to the implant also differs—through a camera or via infrared signals that come from a device mounted on lens frames. The chip will (if successful) treat retinitis pigmentosa and macular degeneration.

Currently computer software is helping restore some sight to the legally blind. Software developed in France can calculate the dimensions for glasses that will maximize the amount of light transmitted to any part of the retina that is still functioning. The program calculates the location and size of the portion of the retina that is still working and the level of magnification necessary to restore sight. Using the program has led to a 50 percent improvement in vision. This improvement means that someone who was blind can walk without the aid of a cane or dog.

Computer technology is also helping people who are hearing impaired. A digital hearing aid (essentially a tiny computer), which can be programmed to meet individual needs and adjust to background noise, became available in 1996. Although it cannot help the profoundly deaf, many people found it better at picking up faint sounds than older models. Digital technology has also made possible the development of the cochlear implant (cleared by the FDA in 1996), a device that has been shown to be of some benefit to hearing-impaired people with intact auditory nerves. The device consists of an internal element surgically implanted behind the ear and a small computer that can be carried. The computer, which is a speech processor, digitizes sound. It is attached to the implant by a cord. The computer sends the digitized code to the implant and then to the inner ear where it is interpreted as sound. Although called an implant, because of its size, most of it is not actually implanted. The size is needed to accommodate the power needs of translating analog to digital signals. However, in 2003, a researcher from Massachusetts Institute of Technology began working on a low-power analog device that would be fully implanted.

One of the problems of hearing aids is that they may amplify sound, but do not indicate where the sound is coming from. Researchers in Sweden are creating a system that includes microphones in eyeglasses. When the sound is heard, it is analyzed by a computer. Pads in the frames of the glasses will vibrate, telling the user where the sound originated.

CFES TECHNOLOGY

Myoectrically controlled prostheses, you recall, use the electrical impulses transmitted by muscles to stimulate movement in artificial limbs. **Computerized functional electrical stimulation (CFES or FES)** directly applies low-level electrical stimulation to muscles that cannot receive these signals from the brain. CFES technology was originally developed by NASA. FES has been used for many years in pacemakers and other implanted devices. It is now used to strengthen paralyzed muscles with exercise. It can be used to simulate a full cardiovascular workout for people who are paralyzed, reducing the secondary effects of paralysis. FES even makes it possible to restore movement to some limbs paralyzed by stroke and spinal injury. By stimulating the correct muscles, people who are paralyzed can walk. The amount of electricity is controlled by a microprocessor, which uses feedback from the body to adjust itself.

A normal arm or leg moves because a specific muscle contracts in response to an electrical signal from the brain. A spinal cord injury can prevent these signals from traveling between the brain and any muscle below the injury. Although the muscles still have the ability to move, they do not receive the necessary signals. FES stimulates the muscles directly, sending the electrical signals using electrodes on the skin's surface. On April 1, 2003, Medicare began covering the Parastep system, one of the systems using FES that allows paraplegics to walk. In 2002 the National Institutes of Health gave a $3.1 million grant to the University of Delaware's Center for Biomedical Engineering to develop a system using FES and robots that will assist paralyzed stroke patients. The robot will help move the patient's legs to teach him or her to walk. They hope to develop an FES device that is small and wearable.

FES is used in many implanted medical devices, some of which we have come to take for granted. Computers delivering electrical stimulation to the heart are permanently embedded in the human body as pacemakers. A more advanced pacemaker, based on two-way communications technology developed by NASA, allows the doctor to regulate the pacemaker from outside the patient's body, even via the Internet. More complicated than a pacemaker, an implantable cardioverter defibrillator monitors heart rate and gives a jolt of electricity when needed. According to the FDA, in a clinical study it restored normal heart rate in 91 percent of the patients. Devices are being tested and approved constantly. In September 1997, the FDA approved an implanted neural prosthesis that will restore some hand movement to quadriplegics. It "allows people with paraplegia to grasp, hold, and release objects by electrically stimulating their muscles. The Freehand system is the world's first surgically implanted device approved by the FDA to restore movement to a paralyzed limb" (FDA Approves Neural Prosthesis, 1997). After a period of training, the device enabled quadriplegics to feed themselves and hold a pen. In March 1998 the FDA approved a breathing pacemaker. It controls breathing by sending electrical impulses to the phrenic nerve.

In July 1997, the FDA approved an implanted device that reduces seizures in people with epilepsy by delivering electrical signals to the brain. Implanted pacemakers (Activa) for the brain are also used to help control the tremors of Parkinson's. This device has wires that connect to the electrodes in the brain. Pacemakers for the brain are being tested for treatment of bipolar disorder and depression. Research is being done on the use of implanted computerized devices to predict and prevent seizures. Bluetooth technology makes it possible for computerized devices to be linked, so that when a pacemaker senses a heart attack, a cell phone will dial 911.

RISKS POSED BY IMPLANTS

Many of the developments we have mentioned in this chapter involve surgically implanting chips or mechanical devices in human beings. These include heart pacemakers, neural implants, drug delivery systems, and some devices under development, like the retinal implant. Although millions of people are walking around with implants, we should remember that implants pose some risks, including rejection of the implant and infection at the site. Some implants can cause blood clots and require the user to take anticlotting medications. Research is currently being done to lower the risks of implants. Some scientists are focusing on creating more user-friendly materials that the human body will accept. Research is beginning at Rensselaer Polytechnic Institute in New York. Using a technique called microdialysis, the project will attempt to look at the body's response to an implant at the cellular level. A tiny probe would take a sample of fluid at the point where the implant and body meet. The analysis of this fluid can show early signs of rejection or infection.

CONCLUSION

Information technology has made possible major improvements in medical devices. This chapter could not be an exhaustive survey since new devices are being developed and approved every year. Computerized monitors (whether stand-alone or networked) can continuously collect data from patients, notifying hospital personnel of a change. Adaptive technology will continue to improve the quality of life of people with disabilities. Assistive devices make it possible for people who are physically challenged to work and live independently. Computerized prostheses have been developed that work almost as well as natural limbs. FES is used in implanted devices, such as pacemakers, and to restore movement to paralyzed limbs.

SELECTED READINGS

Linda Carroll. "Doctors Look Ahead to 'Pacemakers for the Brain.'" *New York Times,* February 18, 2003.

Anne Eisenberg. "Beyond Voice Recognition, to a Computer That Reads Lips." *New York Times,* September 11, 2003.

IN THE NEWS

Doctors Look Ahead to "Pacemakers for the Brain"

by Linda Carroll

While some scientists try to tease out the mechanics of susceptibility to seizures, others seek ways to predict them and head them off.

Aided by smaller and faster computers, researchers say they will soon be able to predict seizures and to design tiny implantable devices that will interrupt them with jolts of electricity or tiny squirts of medication directly into the brain.

Until recently, scientists thought that seizures came on suddenly, with no warning. But new research has shown that seizures start with a tiny spark of activity and that they take hours to build to a surge.

"Seizures develop over time," said Dr. Brian Litt, an assistant professor of neurology at the University of Pennsylvania. "They don't just strike you like lightning."

After researchers realized how slowly seizures developed, they decided to study recordings of brain waves, electroencephalographs, to see whether they could discern any precursors.

As it turns out, scientists had a ready source of EEGs that had been gathered from epilepsy patients who went to hospitals for surgery.

All of the patients scheduled for surgery to remove damaged, seizing brain tissues have their brain waves recorded for several days.

When researchers looked at these recordings with standard analyses, they could not find any warning signs before seizures.

Then the scientists started using methods that are derived from chaos theory, and the seizure patterns started to become clear.

In December, researchers from Arizona State University showed that they could predict more than 80 percent of seizures with a computer program using chaos theory that analyzed brain waves.

On average, warnings of impending surges occurred more than an hour before the seizure, said Dr. Leon D. Iasemidis, an associate professor of bioengineering.

The process is not perfect, though. The computer periodically issued false alarms.

Such research could eventually lead to a "cure" for seizures, Dr. Iasemidis said, adding, "We envision a device that would automatically release a very low dose of an anti-epilepsy drug or an electrical signal that would block the seizure."

Dr. Litt and Dr. Iasemidis said "pacemakers for the brain" were a few years away.

Dr. Litt added: "Devices that react to the electrical start of a seizure, before the onset of overt clinical symptoms, are actually in early testing in humans now.

"But they have a fair amount of development to go. Devices to predict the onset and then trigger therapy are likely a few years away."

IN THE NEWS

What's Next: Beyond Voice Recognition, to a Computer That Reads Lips

by Anne Eisenberg

Personal computers have changed a lot in the last few decades, but not in the way that people communicate with them. Typing on a keyboard, with the help of a mouse, remains the most common interface.

But pounding away at a set of keys is hard on the hands and tethers users to the keyboard. Automatic speech recognition offers some relief—the systems work reasonably well for office dictation, for instance. But voice recognition is not effective in noisy places like cars, train stations or the corner cash machine, and it may stumble even under the best of conditions. Humans are still much better than any computer at the subtleties of speech recognition.

But teaching computers to read lips might boost the accuracy of automatic speech recognition. Listeners naturally use mouth movements to help them understand the difference between "bat" and "pat," for instance. If distinctions like this could be added to a computer's databank with the aid of cheap cameras and powerful processors, speech recognition software might work a lot better, even in noisy places.

Scientists at I.B.M.'s research center in Westchester County, at Intel's centers in China and California and in many other labs are developing just such digital lip-reading systems to augment the accuracy of speech recognition.

Chalapathy Neti, a senior researcher at I.B.M.'s Thomas J. Watson Research Center in Yorktown Heights, N.Y., has spent the past four years focusing on how to boost the performance of speech recognition with cameras. Dr. Neti manages the center's research in audiovisual speech technologies. "We humans fuse audio and visual perception in deciding what is being spoken," he said. A computer, he said, can be trained to do this job, too.

At I.B.M., the process starts by getting the computer and camera to locate the person who is speaking, searching for skin-tone pixels, for instance, and then using statistical models that detect any object in that area that resembles a face. Then, with the face in view, vision algorithms focus on the mouth region, estimating the location of many features, including the corners and center of the lips.

If the camera looked solely at the mouth, though, only about 12 to 14 sounds could be distinguished visually, Dr. Neti said—for instance, the difference between the explosive initial "p" and its close relative "b." So the group enlarged the visual region to include many types of movements. "We tried using additional visible articulators like jaw movements and the lower cheek, and other movements of tongue and teeth," he said, "and that turned out to be beneficial." Then the visual and audio features were combined and analyzed by statistical models that predicted what the speaker was saying.

CHAPTER SUMMARY

This chapter introduced the reader to the uses of digital technology in medical instruments, adaptive devices, and prostheses, and to the use of FES technology.

- Computerized medical instruments with embedded microprocessors are used to monitor patients and administer medication.
  - Computerized drug delivery systems are programmable and can detect incorrect flow.
  - Computerized monitoring devices include physiological monitoring systems, arrhythmia monitors, pulmonary monitors, fetal monitors, and neonatal monitoring systems. They continuously monitor a patient's condition and can be programmed to sound an alarm and notify personnel of a dangerous change.
  - Some monitors are part of a network; this makes it possible to check the patient's condition from a central location, and can decrease response time in emergencies.
- Information technology has had a tremendous impact on people with disabilities.
- The Americans with Disabilities Act of 1990 requires employers to provide "reasonable accommodation" for people with disabilities on the job. Digital technology has made this possible.
  - Speech recognition technology allows people without sight or without the use of their hands to interact with computers. Other special input devices include head mice and puff straws.
  - Page scanners, speech synthesizers, and screen readers enable the computer to speak to you if you cannot see the screen, and for you if you cannot speak.
  - Speech recognition can also be used to control appliances in the home, allowing disabled people to live independently.
- Prostheses are artificial replacement limbs and organs.
  - Myoelectric limbs contain a microchip and motor and respond to contractions of the muscle of the natural limb. They work almost as well as natural limbs.
  - CAD/CAM is used in the design and manufacture of prosthetic limbs.
  - Computer technology has contributed to the development of a prosthetic hand whose fingers can be separately controlled and prostheses, which will sense hot and cold.
  - Computer technology is also contributing to developments, which help restore hearing and sight.
- Computerized functional electrical stimulation delivers low-level electrical stimulation to muscles.
- It is used in implanted devices such as pacemakers and to stimulate paralyzed muscles, even enabling the paralyzed to walk.
- Implants pose the risk of infection and rejection.

KEY TERMS

adaptive technology
Americans with
  Disabilities Act
  of 1990
arrhythmia monitors
assistive technology
augmentative communi-
  cation device
biomicroscopes
computerized functional
  electrical stimula-
  tion (CFES or FES)
computerized medical
  instruments
continuous speech
  recognition systems

corneal topography
discrete speech recog-
  nition systems
environmental control
  systems
fetal monitors
GDx Access Optical
  biometry
head mouse
Heidelberg Retinal
  Tomograph (HRT)
myoelectric
neonatal monitors
optical biometry
Optomap Panoramic200
page scanners

physiological monitoring
  systems
prosthetic devices
puff straws
pulmonary monitors
screen reader software
speaker-dependent
speaker-independent
speech recognition
speech synthesizers
text telephone
tonometers
Tracey Visual Function
  Analyzer

REVIEW QUESTIONS

Multiple Choice

1. Computerized medical devices have some advantages over their predecessors. Among them are _____.
   A. No human intervention is required.
   B. No necessity for programming.
   C. They can be programmed to detect values outside of a certain range and sound an alarm.
   D. None of the above

2. Networked devices _____.
   A. Can reduce response time in emergencies
   B. Are most often found in ERs, CCUs, and ICUs
   C. Can display findings in a central location
   D. All of the above

3. Puff straws, head mice, and speech recognition software could be characterized as _____.
   A. Prosthetic devices
   B. Assistive devices
   C. Adaptive devices
   D. B or C

4. A _____ digitizes printed text so that it can be input.
   A. Page scanner
   B. Speech synthesizer
   C. Screen reader
   D. Speech recognition system
5. _____ is an alternate input device that a blind person could use.
   A. Braille keyboard
   B. Speech recognition software
   C. A or B
   D. Screen reader
6. CFES technology was first developed by _____.
   A. NASA
   B. Department of Defense
   C. National Institute of Health
   D. University of Pennsylvania
7. CFES delivers low-level electrical stimulation and is used _____.
   A. In pacemakers
   B. To simulate workouts for paralyzed muscles
   C. To restore movement to paralyzed muscles
   D. All of the above
8. The _____ restores some measure of hearing to deaf people with intact auditory nerves.
   A. Artificial ear
   B. Cochlear implant
   C. Hearing pacemaker
   D. Prosthetic ear
9. Prosthetic limbs, which contain motors and respond to signals transmitted by the muscles in the residual limb, are called _____.
   A. Energy-storing limbs
   B. Myoelectric limbs
   C. Computerized limbs
   D. Motorized limbs
10. Discrimination against people with disabilities is prohibited by the _____.
    A. Civil Rights Act
    B. Fourteenth Amendment to the U.S. Constitution
    C. Americans with Disabilities Act
    D. None of the above

True/False Questions

1. It is possible to control the mouse pointer with brain waves. _____
2. Computer software can help restore some sight to people who are legally blind. _____
3. Hardware and software exist that will allow you to control your home environment by giving voice commands. _____
4. Myoelectric limbs are made possible by computers. _____

5. Currently, an artificial eye can restore sight to the blind. _____
6. Discrete speech recognition systems require more memory than continuous speech recognition systems. _____
7. Implanted pacemakers for the brain are used to help control the tremors of Parkinson's. _____
8. Networked devices can interact with each other. _____
9. Computerized cardiac monitors cannot distinguish between cardiac arrest and a wire coming loose. _____
10. Speech recognition software can understand whatever you say. _____.

Critical Thinking

1. Evaluate you work space at home, school, or work. How would you design an adaptive environment for people who are mobility impaired?
2. How would you design an adaptive environment for people with speech impairments?
3. How would you design an adaptive environment for people who are blind?
4. The quality of life can be greatly enhanced with the extraordinary CFES technology and advances in prosthetic devices. However, the present cost to the patient can be prohibitive. How would you make this technology available to anyone who needs it?
5. How will the health care professions be affected by all the computerized and technical advances concerning disabilities?

SOURCES

Anderson, Annalee. "Language Learning Using Infrared Toys." 2003 Conference Proceedings. csun.edu (2003; June 10, 2003).

Anderson, Sandra. *Computer Literacy for Health Care Professionals.* New York: Delmar, 1992.

Berck, Judith. "Tools for Blind Students." *New York Times,* August 6, 1996, pp. 16, 27.

Bhattacharjee, Yudhijit. "Smart Wheelchairs Will Ease Many Paths." nyt.com, (May 10, 2001; June 18, 2003).

———. "So That's Who's Talking: A Hearing Aid Points to the Sound." nyt.com (September 27, 2001; September 28, 2001).

Carroll, Linda. "Doctors Look Ahead to 'Pacemakers for the Brain.'" nyt.com (February 18, 2003; June 10, 2003).

Cefalu, William T., and William Weir. "New Technologies in Diabetes Care." patientcareonline.com (September 2003; October 24, 2003).

"Cochlear Implants." nidcd.nih.gov (May 13, 2003; June 12, 2003).

"Computerized Prosthetics." www.apta.org (2003; June 15, 2003).

Conference and Preconference Papers and Workshops. October 16–18, 2003. closingthegap.com/conf (October 16, 2003; October 14, 2003).

Coughlin, Kevin. "Program Gives Disabled a Helping Hand." *Star-Ledger,* February 23, 1998, p. 1, 25.

"Early Infection and Rejection Detection: Microdialysis Technique May Help Implants Stay Longer." rpi.edu (July 28, 2003; October 24, 2003).

Eisenberg, Anne. "Analog over Digital? For a Better Ear Implant, Yes." nyt.com (May 29, 2003; June 12, 2003).

———. "Beyond Voice Recognition, to a Computer That Reads Lips." nyt.com (September 11, 2003; October 24, 2003).

———. "A Chip That Mimics a Retina but Strains for Light." nyt.com (August 9, 2001; August 30, 2002).

———. "A Gaze That Dictates, with Intuitive Software as the Scribe." nyt.com (September 12, 2002; September 12, 2002).

———. "The Kind of Noise That Keeps a Body on Balance." nyt.com (November 14, 2002; June 10, 2003).

———. "What's Next: A Chip That Mimics Neurons, Firing Up the Memory." nyt.com (June 2, 2002; October 11, 2003).

———. "What's Next: Glasses So Smart They Know What You're Looking At." nyt.com (June 28, 2001; August 30, 2002).

———. "When the Athlete's Heart Falters, a Monitor Dials for Help." nyt.com, (2002; June 10, 2003).

"Environmental Control Systems for People With Spinal Cord Injuries." www.abilitycorp.com (1999; June 10, 2003).

"FDA Approves New Glucose Test for Adult Diabetics." *FDA News.* www.fda.gov (March 22, 2001; June 11, 2003).

"FDA Approves Neural Prosthesis." http://www.cwru.edu/pubaff/univcomm/cwru1097.htm#freehand (September 1997; May 17, 2004).

Felton, Bruce. "Technologies That Enable the Disabled." *New York Times,* September 14, 1997, pp. BU1, BU10.

Flynn, Karen, Liz Adams, and Elaine Alligood. "VA Technology Assessment Short Report—Computerized Lower Limb Prosthesis." www.va.gov (March 2000; June 15, 2003).

Gallagher, David. "For the Errant Heart, a Chip That Packs a Wallop." nyt.com (August 16, 2001; August 17, 2001).

Glassman, Mark. "A Braille Phone Organizer Connects the Dots and the User." nyt.com (April 17, 2003; April 18, 2003).

Grady, Denise. "Digital Hearing Aids Hold New Promise." *New York Times,* June 4, 1997.

Happ, Mary. "Feasibility of an Augmentative Device for Head and Neck Cancer Patients." pitt.edu (May 15, 2002; June 10, 2003).

———. "Feasibility Study of an Augmentative Communication Device with Temporarily Voiceless Patients in Critical Care." pitt.edu (January 31, 2001; June 10, 2003).

Henkel, John. "Parkinson's Disease: New Treatments Slow Onslaught of Symptoms." US FDA. www.fda.gov (1998; June 10, 2003).

Humphrey, Jonathan. "Computerized Leg Gives Ex-bouncer His Bounce Back." MaineToday.com (December 2, 2002; June 15, 2003).

Junker, Andrew H. "A Revolutionary Approach to Computer Access: Coherent Detected Periodic Brainwave Computer Control." Brainfingers.com (2003; June 10, 2003).

Krieg, Lawrence. "Introduction to Computerized Medical Instrumentation." courses.wccnet.edu (November 7, 2001; June 12, 2003).

Lazzaro, John. *Adaptive Technologies for Learning and Work Environments.* Chicago: American Library Association, 1993.

Marriott, Michel. "With Wires, the Disabled Gain Control." nyt.com (April 27, 2003; April 27, 2003).

"Medicare at Last! Medicare Coverage of AAC Devices Is Now in Effect." www.ncds.org/
    kornreich/at_info/McareUpdate.htm www.ncds.org/kornreich/at_info/
    McareUpdate.htm (2002; June 10, 2003).

"Medicare to Pay for FES Walking System." www.paralysis.org (2002; February 3, 2003).

New Device Approval GlucoWatch® Automatic Glucose Biographer. www.fda.gov (March 22,
    2001; June 11, 2003).

New Device Approval Medtronic Model 7250 Jewel® AF Implantable Cardioverter
    Defibrillator System—P980050/S1. www.fda.gov (April 1, 2001; June 10, 2003).

"New, Light Prosthetics Helping Amputees Function Better." wnbc.com (June 12, 2003;
    June 18, 2003).

Norwood, Robert. "NASA Technologies Contribute to Medical Breakthroughs." *Advanced
    Technologies* (March–April 1998).

Nussbaum, Debra. "Bringing the Visual World of the Web to the Blind." *New York Times,*
    March 26, 1998, p. G8.

Ouellette, Jennifer. "Biomaterials Facilitate Medical Breakthroughs." American Institute of
    Physics. www.aip.org (October/November 2001; October 24, 2003).

"Pacemaker for the Brain." Southwestern Medical Center. http://www3.utsouthwestern
    .edu/library/consumer/brainPaceMkr.htm (January 7, 2002; June 10, 2003).

"Pacemaker for the Brain." WGBH.com (January 24, 2002; June 10, 2003).

"'Pacemaker for the Brain' May Offer Hope to Sufferers of Severe Parkinson's Disease."
    Penn State University. www.sciencedaily.com/releases/2001/12/011224084212.htm
    (December 27, 2001; June 10, 2003).

"Quadriplegia: Neural Prosthesis for Grasping Okayed." *Physicians Weekly* 14, no. 36
    (September 22, 1997). physweekly.com (September 22, 1997; June 11, 2003).

Rachkesperger, Tracy. "Growing Up with AAC." asha.org (2002; June 10, 2003).

RehabEngineer. "Augmentative Communications." rehabengineer.homestead.com
    (October 20, 2001; June 12, 2003).

Roberts, Dan. "Microchip Implantation." www.mdsupport.org (October 2002; October 24,
    2003).

Senn, Jim. *Information Technology in Business: Principles, Practices, and Opportunities,* 2d ed.
    Upper Saddle River, NJ: Prentice-Hall, 1998.

Smith, Graeme. "Environmental Control Systems for People with Spinal Cord Injuries."
    www.abilitycorp.com (September 1999; May 9, 2004).

Spectrum Eye Care. infospectrumeyecare.com (January 19, 2003; January 14, 2004).

Stresing, Diane. "Digital Implants Dig In." *Laptop* (November 2002): 90–96.

Taub, Eric. "Typing with Two Hands, No Fingers." nyt.com (2003; May 2, 2003).

"$3.1 Million NIH Grant Funds Research to Help Stroke Patients." *University of Delaware
    Daily.* www.udel.edu/PR/UDaily/01-02/NIHgrant101702.html (October 17, 2002;
    June 12, 2003).

Weingarten, Marc. "For an Irregular Lens, an Optical Blueprint." nyt.com (September 12,
    2002).

Wiener, Jon. "USC Ophthalmologists Announce Launch of Permanent Retinal Implant
    Study." hsc.usc.edu (April 30, 2002; June 11, 2003).

Wilson, Maryann. "Computerized Prosthetics." *PT Magazine,* December 1, 2001.
    http://www.apta.org/PTmagazine/Current_Issue?&id[1]=19238#19691 (2003;
    June 12, 2003).

"What Is an Insulin Pump? How Does It Work?" http://www.minimed.com (2003; June 12,
    2003).

CHAPTER 10

Informational Resources:
Computer-Assisted Instruction, Expert Systems, and Health Information Online

OUTLINE

- **Learning Objectives**
- **Overview**
- **Education**
  - *The Visible Human*
  - *Computer-Assisted Instruction*
  - *Simulation Software*
  - *Virtual Reality Simulations*
  - *Patient Simulators*
  - *Distance Learning*
- **Decision Support: Expert Systems**
- **Health Information on the Internet**
  - *Medical Literature Databases*
  - *E-mail*
  - *Self-help on the Web*
  - *Support Groups on the Web*
  - *Judging the Reliability of Health Information on the Internet*
- **Self-help Software**
- **Conclusion**
- **Selected Reading**
- **Chapter Summary**
- **Key Terms**
- **Review Questions**
  - *Multiple Choice*
  - *True/False Questions*
  - *Critical Thinking*
- **Sources**
- **Related Web Sites**

LEARNING OBJECTIVES

Upon completion of this chapter, you will be able to

- List the many informational resources that computer technology and the Internet have made available and their use in the health care fields.
- Describe the use of computer-assisted instruction in health care education.
- Discuss the Visible Human Project; many simulation programs use data from this project.
- Describe simulation programs such as ADAM, which make use of text and graphics.
- Describe simulation programs that make use of virtual reality to teach surgical procedures, dentistry, and other skills.
- Define patient simulators.
- Be aware of the existence of distance learning programs in health care education.
- Discuss the role of expert systems, such as INTERNIST, MYCIN, and POEMS in health care.
- Describe the resources on the Internet, including medical literature databases, physicians' use of e-mail, general information and misinformation, and support groups, and be able to discuss both the positive and negative consequences of using the Internet as a resource for health information.
- Discuss the availability of self-help software.

OVERVIEW

Computers and the Internet have made increasing amounts of information available to more people than in the past and have changed the way we teach and learn in many fields. Health care is no exception. Software exists to teach both providers and consumers of health care. The Internet makes vast stores of information available to patients and health care providers and can provide support for people with various illnesses. Self-help programs present information for consumers of health care. Databases, such as MEDLINE, and expert systems, such as MYCIN and INTERNIST, make the latest medical research easily available to health care professionals. The existence of these new informational resources has made it possible for health care professionals to learn in a variety of environments, via distance learning. These same developments have made it necessary for health care providers to be computer literate in order to take advantage of new and expanding sources of information.

EDUCATION

The Visible Human

The **Visible Human Project** is a computerized library of human anatomy at the National Library of Medicine. It began in 1986; it is an ongoing project. It has created "complete, anatomically detailed, three-dimensional representations of the male and female human body" (Visible Human Project, 2003). The images are accessible over the Internet. Hundreds of people have used these images on computer screens where they can be rotated and flipped, taken apart and put back together. Structures can be enlarged and highlighted. The images, also available on CD-ROM, have been used by students of anatomy, researchers, surgeons, and dentists who discovered a new face muscle. There is some speculation that the Visible Human's virtual cadavers may replace actual cadavers in medical education. The Visible Human is available for both teaching and research. ADAM, a program that is used to teach anatomy, uses data from the Visible Human. The data provided by the Visible Human is the source for a virtual colonoscopy.

The National Library of Medicine is moving the project "From Data to Knowledge." Some current aspects of the Visible Human will allow users to *see* and *feel* anatomic flythroughs on the Web and to see surrounding structures. Students can use a wand to create three-dimensional structures from two-dimensional structures or from segmented slices. Students will be able to build and palpate organs. An **explorable virtual human** is being developed. It will include authoring tools that engineers can use to build anatomical models that will allow students to experience how real anatomical structures feel, appear, and sound.

A new project called the **virtual human embryo** is digitizing some of the 7,000 human embryos lost in miscarriages, which have been kept by the National Museum of Health and Medicine of the Armed Forces Institute of Pathology since the 1880s. An embryo develops in 23 stages over the first eight weeks of pregnancy. The project will include at least one embryo from each stage. It will be sectioned and sliced. Each slice will be placed under a microscope, and digital images will be created. Users will be able to access the images on DVDs and CDs, and manipulate and study them.

Computer-Assisted Instruction

Computer-assisted instruction (CAI) is used at all stages of the educational process. Drill-and-practice software is used to teach skills that require memorization. Simulation software simulates a complex process. The student is presented with a situation and given choices. The student is then shown what affect that choice would have on the situation. Early simulation programs used text and graphics to describe a situation. Later, animation and sound were added. Today, some programs use virtual reality so that the student actually feels as if he or she were there.

What is the effect of CAI on education for health care professionals? A quantitative analysis was performed of 47 studies of the use of CAI in the health science professions in 1992. The studies all compared student performance in CAI with traditional teaching methods. Thirty-two of the studies concluded that CAI is superior. However, the analysis of the studies also concluded that some of the 47 studies jumped to conclusions that were unsupported by the data they collected. The statistical analysis concludes that CAI does have a "moderate-sized effect." A later review of literature on CAI found that computers are having "little effect on health care education." However, it was found to be a helpful supplement in some areas of study.

Simulation Software

Simulation programs have been used for many years in nursing education. As early as 1963, computer-based nursing courses were developed using **PLATO (Programmed Logic for Automatic Teaching Operations)**. The student sat before her or his "television screen and . . . electronic keyset similar to . . . a standard typewriter" (Bitzer, 1982) and was presented with hypothetical patients to evaluate, problems to solve, and questions to answer. The program used both text and graphics. It was judged to be successful in allowing students to progress at their own pace and in their own style of learning. At that time, most schools did not have the computers necessary to use these programs. Now computers are used throughout the educational system, and simulation programs are a taken-for-granted part of health care education. Programs such as **ILIAD** have been used for years and provide hypothetical cases for the student to evaluate. The student's diagnostic abilities are then compared with the computer's. **ADAM** teaches anatomy and physiology. It uses two- and three-dimensional images (some of them created from the Visible Human data) and has versions available for both patients and professionals. It is interactive, allowing the user to click away over 100 layers of the body and see more than 4000 structures! Using multiple windows, the user can compare different views of one anatomical structure. A program called eXpert Trainer helps students learn the skills needed for minimally invasive surgery (see Chapter 7).

Virtual Reality Simulations

The newest simulations use virtual reality techniques, requiring the power of supercomputers. Simulations using virtual reality can make health care education safer and more effective (Figure 10.1). These simulations are particularly useful in teaching procedures that are guided by *haptic* clues (sense of feel) and where a mistake can seriously harm a patient. Now, before a medical resident operates on a live patient, surgery can be simulated. Students can manipulate surgical instruments while watching a computer monitor. Motors in the instruments provide resistance so that the student learns how much pressure is required for a particular task. Using a device developed by Dr. Thomas Krummel, of the Penn State College of Medicine, the student can "actually feel . . . [the tissue] . . . as the needle goes through" (Wilson, 1997). Dr. Krummel has developed another device using a mannequin and computer imaging, which allows medical students to practice inserting a bronchoscope into a child's trachea. Dr. Krummel has also designed a program to teach surgical skills to new students at Penn State. The school uses a four-step program, which first teaches skills; then uses a 3-D anatomical program. The third step is to perform the tasks learned while monitored by a computer. The last step involves performing the operation on a simulator that mimics the human body and its responses.

Virtual reality simulations are also being used to train surgeons to perform minimally invasive operations. Because the surgeon operates in a restricted field, which she or he cannot directly see, MIS requires extensive training. One MIS trainer (called **KISMET**) uses "a rough imitation of the . . . abdomen. . . . The trainee [is provided]

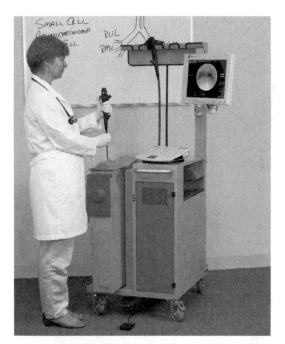

(a)

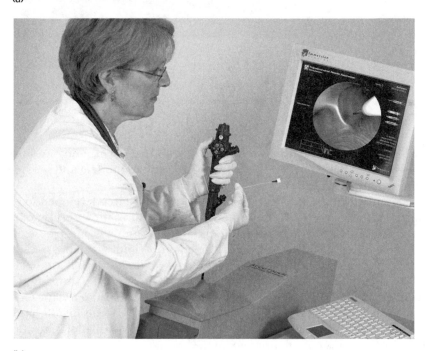

(b)

FIGURE 10.1 Simulations of procedures created by Immersion help students learn procedures such as bronchoscopies (a) and (b).

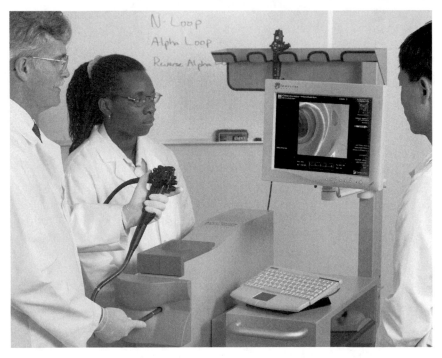

(c)

FIGURE 10.1   *(continued)*   (c) Simulation of a colonoscopy procedure.
Reproduced by the permission of Immersion Corporation. Copyright © 2004 Immersion
Corporation. All rights reserved.

with a virtual operation area and a real-time 'synthetic' endoscopic view"
(Versweyveld, 1998). KISMET also allows the student to feel and see how soft tissue
reacts to grasping and cutting in real time.

Simulations using virtual reality are currently being developed to teach the administration of an epidural anesthetic, which requires the insertion of a catheter in
the epidural space of the spinal column; the only guide is one's sense of feel. A mistake could leave a patient paralyzed. The epidural simulator allows the student to perform the procedure while feeling the resistance of the tissue, but without endangering
a live patient. Students can learn to administer an IV from a simulation program instead of practicing on a rubber arm. "The student is able to sense the tactile response
of needle and catheter insertion—from the 'pop' as the needle enters the skin
through entry into the vein lumen" (Hensley, 1999). Simulations are also being used
to help teach surgeons to operate on the prostate. As minimally invasive surgery becomes more common, virtual reality simulators that mimic the sights, sounds, and feel
of these procedures are being further developed.

In dentistry, virtual reality simulations make use of mannequins to allow students
to practice filling cavities while watching both the mannequin and a monitor. The

student feels the tooth via the instruments, learning to distinguish between a healthy and a diseased tooth. The student's work is immediately evaluated. The procedure can be repeated numerous times.

In 2002, researchers created the virtual stomach, a computer simulation. The stomach can be used to study how medications and nutrients decompose and are dispersed. Using the virtual stomach has already led to new knowledge: tablets break down at the bottom of the stomach, and density of tablets is important to the speed with which they break down.

Patient Simulators

Human patient simulators are programmable mannequins on which students can practice medical procedures (Figure 10.2). The simulator has liquids flowing through its blood vessels, inhales oxygen and exhales carbon dioxide, produces heart and lung sounds, has eyes that open and close, pupils that dilate, a tongue that can swell to simulate an allergic reaction. The student can perform an electrocardiogram, take the pulse, and measure blood pressure and temperature. Medications can be administered intravenously; the mannequin reads the bar code and reacts as it has been programmed to react. Students can practice intubations and needle decompression of pneumothorax (accumulation of air or gas in the lung); chest tubes may be inserted. Different types of patients can be simulated, including a healthy adult, a woman experiencing problems with pregnancy, and a middle-aged man suffering from hypertension. Another mannequin, called **PediaSim** is a virtual child. It can be programmed also, for instance, to have an allergic reaction to peanuts.

These mannequins can be used in classrooms or in simulated emergency situations. A crowded corner of an emergency room can be simulated, with noise, time limits, and physical constraints for the student. This brings the simulation even closer to reality.

Distance Learning

The expansion of information and telecommunications technology has made it possible to learn in a variety of settings—not just the traditional classroom. Distance learning refers to learning in an environment where student and instructor are not physically face-to-face. It may mean anything from simply picking up assignments on the Internet and e-mailing a paper to a professor, to a complete videoconference system where teacher and students see and hear each other via cameras, monitors, and microphones. Distance learning for health care professionals usually falls somewhere in between. A course may use Internet resources, videotapes, and CD-ROMs, along with traditional textbooks and other printed material. Both health science institutions and the government have made educational resources available over the Internet. Through the Learning Center for Interactive Technology, the National Library of Medicine's Cognitive Science Branch provides links to databases, information, and tutorials for health care professionals, making it possible for them to continue learning wherever there is a computer with a link to the Internet. The National

FIGURE 10.2   Human Patient Simulators™ HPS® made by METI® give students practice on virtual adults and children in realistic situations such as the OR and ICU. (a) PediaSim® Pediatric Simulator by METI®. (b) HPS®.
Courtesy of Medical Education Technologies, Inc.

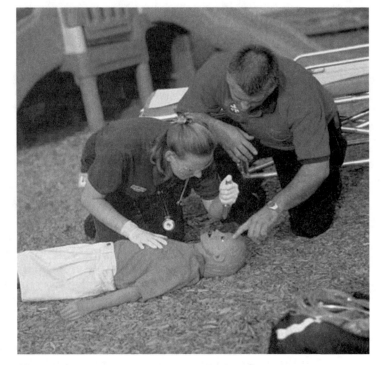

(a)

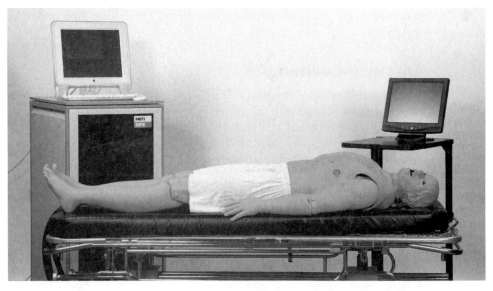

(b)

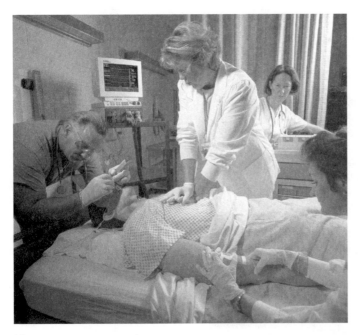

(c)

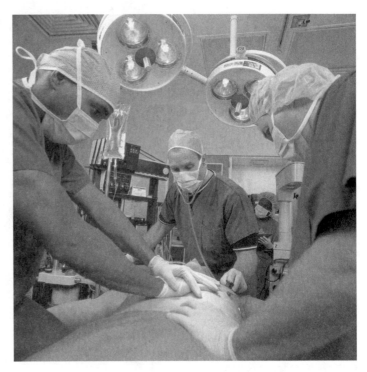

FIGURE 10.2   *(continued)*
(c) HPS® in ICU. (d) HPS in OR®.
Courtesy of Medical Education
Technologies, Inc.

(d)

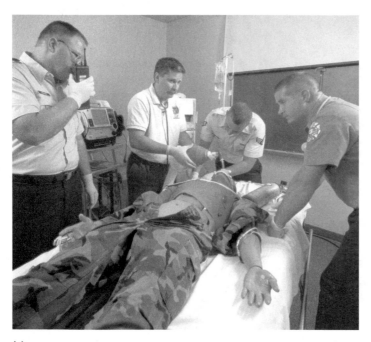

(e)

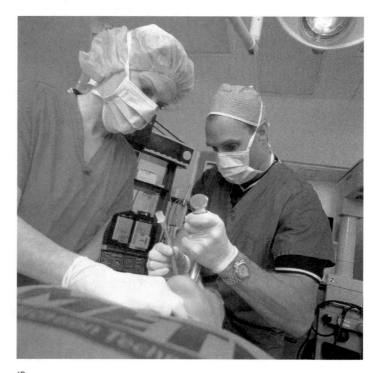

FIGURE 10.2 *(continued)*
(e) and (f) Human Patient
Simulators™ HPS® by METI®
help students learn to perform
procedures.
Courtesy of Medical Education
Technologies, Inc.

(f)

Library of Medicine is also attempting to expand the opportunities for distance learning for health care professionals, and to link existing distance learning sites. Some traditional colleges and universities have degree programs at the graduate and undergraduate level in health sciences that don't require the student to be on campus, but do require self-discipline and access to a computer and the Internet. Public health workers may also learn via distance learning. The **Virtual Hospital** provides online courses for credit for health care professionals.

DECISION SUPPORT: EXPERT SYSTEMS

An expert system is an attempt to make a computer an expert in one narrow field. Both facts and rules about how the facts are used to make decisions in the field are entered in the computer. Expert systems are a branch of artificial intelligence, which examines how computers behave like human beings, that is, in "intelligent" ways. Expert systems have been used in medicine since the 1950s. They are meant to be decision support systems, which help, but do not replace, medical personnel. They are especially useful when there is a limited, well-defined area of knowledge needed for a decision, which will be based on objective data. The doctor enters symptoms, test results, and medical history. The computer either asks for more information or suggests a diagnosis, and perhaps treatment. Some systems give the diagnosis in the form of a probability.

The computer can suggest conditions that the doctor has not thought of since medical school or has simply not considered. However, it is up to the health care professional to confirm the suggestion by tests. Although these systems are very helpful, they have their drawbacks. Each system is an expert in only one limited area. Expert systems may also spend time eliminating conditions that human experts would not even need to consider. However, with the amount of information available today, a computer's ability to organize is crucial.

Studies of diagnostic software have had mixed results. One study of emergency room patients with chest pain found a 97 percent accuracy rate for computers diagnosing heart attacks, to 78 percent for doctors. A study of four programs found them to give correct diagnoses 50 to 75 percent of the time. In 1989, a trial using 31 undiagnosed cases compared the diagnosis of an expert system in the area of Internal Medicine called QMR with the best guess of the attending physician and found the following: the accuracy of the physician was 80 percent compared with 85 percent for the expert system and 60 percent for the house staff.

One early medical expert system was developed at Stanford University in 1970. Called **MYCIN**, it aids in the diagnosis and treatment of bacterial infections. The doctor types in data about the patient's symptoms; the computer asks for more information until it has enough to suggest a diagnosis. The computer then asks about any drug sensitivities the patient might have, so that treatment may be suggested. MYCIN's diagnostic accuracy equals or surpasses that of human specialists. **INTERNIST** is another expert system developed at the University of Pittsburgh. It contains information about 500 diseases and their 2,900 associated symptoms. A newer expert system developed in England is called **Post Operative Expert Medical System (POEMS)**; it focuses on patients who become sick while recovering from surgery. The **Databank for Cardiovascular Disease** at Duke University is a highly specialized expert system that combines computer monitoring with extensive collections of information on cardiac patients.

In October 1998, a review of decision support systems was published in the *Journal of the American Medical Association (JAMA)*. The review looks at studies of the use of some of the systems during the past quarter century. The quality of expert systems varies. However, in certain areas, specifically, drug use and preventive medicine, expert systems contributed positively to the doctor's performance.

HEALTH INFORMATION ON THE INTERNET

Both doctors and consumers who have access to the Internet use it as a source of health care information. Care should be used when searching for health information; the consumer is required to give personal information. This information is being mined for several purposes, including profiling the person most in need of a product or service. Several groups of health care professionals have created a suggested code of conduct for health-related Web sites: They should disclose any information that consumers would find useful, including who has a monetary interest; they should distinguish scientific information from advertising; they should attempt to assure the high quality of information; and they should disclose privacy risks and take steps to ensure privacy. Any health care professional giving advice or other information over the Web should abide by professional standards. The site needs to make it clear to consumers how they can get in touch with the site manager and should encourage feedback.

Some sites, including medical literature databases, are specifically meant for health care professionals. Sixty percent of doctors surveyed said they found Internet information helpful. Many sites are directed to consumers. There are at least 10,000 health-related sites on the Web (excluding support groups). According to the Federal Trade Commission, "consumer online searches for health information are increasing dramatically" (2001 Report to Congress on Telemedicine, 2002). Tens of millions of people log on to the Internet looking for information about medication and disease, suggested cures, and support groups. The Internet (with all of its misinformation) has some reliable sites providing good information.

It should be noted that access to health-related information on the Internet is not equally distributed through society, but is restricted to those with access to computers with an Internet connection and the knowledge to make use of them. The digital divide refers to the gap between information haves and have-nots. White and Asian Americans, those with higher incomes, and higher education are more likely to have computer access and Internet access than low-income, less educated people, and African Americans and Hispanics. People in rural areas have less access to the Internet than people in urban areas. A February 2002 report from the federal government maintained that the digital divide was disappearing quickly. The Bush administration then lowered funding to government programs that supported community-computing centers. However, a 2003 study by sociologist, Dr. Steven Martin at the University of Maryland, concluded that "[c]omputer ownership and Internet use may actually be spreading less quickly among poorer households than among richer households." Between 1998 and 2001, Internet use grew from 14 percent to 25 percent among families with annual incomes of less than $15,000; it grew from 59 percent to 79 percent among families with incomes greater than $75,000. The odds that a poor family would use the Internet grew by a factor of 2.1, while the odds for an affluent family grew by 2.6 percent. Dr. Martin predicts that it will be another 20 years before 90 percent of the poorest quarter of the population owns computers (Guernsey, 2003).

Medical Literature Databases

The capacity of computers to store and organize huge collections of data, to make the data accessible, and to transmit it over telecommunications lines forms the basis of online medical literature databases. The National Library of Medicine provides a collection of 40 computerized databases called **MEDLARS (Medical Literature Analysis and Retrieval System)** containing 18 million references. MEDLARS is available free via the Internet, and can be searched for bibliographical lists or for information (Figure 10.3).

MEDLINE is a comprehensive online database of current medical research, including publications from 1966 to the present containing 8.5 million articles from 3,700 journals. Thirty-one thousand citations are added each month. It has been used in hospitals for years. MEDLINE can be used for academic research or to help a doctor identify a patient's problem. Since MEDLINE is updated daily, it gives access to the most up-to-date information to health care personnel. Although the information in MEDLINE is meant for professionals, 30 percent of its users are patients. **PubMed** is used to search MEDLINE (Figure 10.4). **SDILINE (Selective Dissemination of Information onLINE)** contains only the latest month's additions to MEDLINE. Other MEDLARS databases include AIDSLINE, AIDSTRIALS, and CANCERLIT. DIRLINE is a guide to online information.

In 1998, the National Library of Medicine introduced MEDLINEPlus, which is meant for the general public (Figure 10.5). In 2001 there were 2.3 hits per month. The information is selected using strict guidelines to guarantee accuracy and objectivity.

Databases of drug information are also online. **MediSpan** is a collection of data on drug/drug and drug/food interactions. **Clinical pharmacology** is a database for health care professionals with the latest information on drugs. It also contains information for doctors to distribute to their patients. **New medicines in development** provides information on drugs that have been recently approved and those awaiting approval. **ClinicalTrials.gov** was launched in February 2000; it lists thousands of clinical trials along with their purpose, criteria for participation, location, and contact information (Figure 10.6). **Centerwatch** maintains a Web site that lists 7,000 (of 70,000) current clinical trials in the U.S. Many are recruiting participants. It should

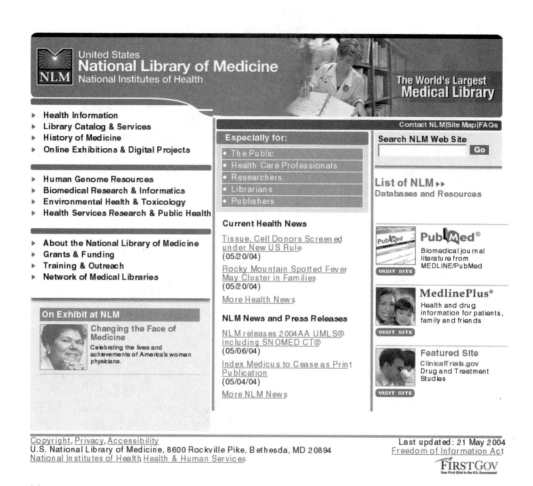

(a)

FIGURE 10.3a and b   The National Library of Medicine maintains many medical literature databases.

be noted, however, that the purpose of drug trials is to test the effectiveness and safety of the medication, not to help those patients participating in the trial. There have been questions raised regarding ethics and adequate safeguards for human subjects who might be drawn in to participating in clinical trials by desperation stemming from illness or poverty. Only one-half of the people who participate in clinical drug trials are actually administered the drug being tested. The other half is given a placebo. Not even the physician knows which patient is receiving which substance. For those interested in the records of drugs that are already on the market, the U.S. FDA's Center for Drug Evaluation and Research maintains a site that provides information on the safety records of drugs and on drug companies and ad campaigns.

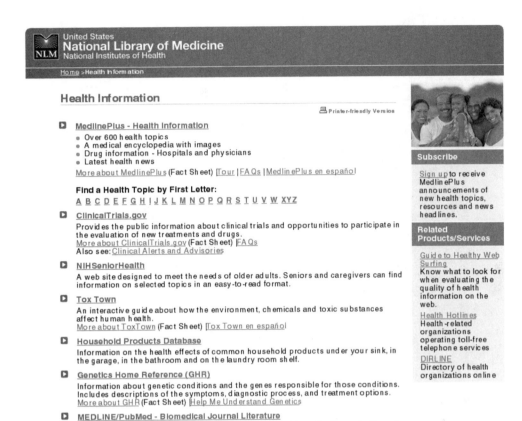

(b)

CINAHL (The Cumulative Index to Nursing and Allied Health Literature) is a database specifically geared to nurses and allied health professionals. It indexes more than 1,200 publications.

Although the existence of these resources is widely known, the effect of their use is not. A review of the literature on the use and effectiveness of electronic information retrieval systems was published in *JAMA* in October 1998. The study found that use is limited. Later studies, however, found that "clinical decision support systems may provide significant benefits in . . . care" (Trowbridge, nd).

E-mail

A majority of health care consumers who go online to search for advice would prefer information from their own doctors online. Many patients want to establish an e-mail con-

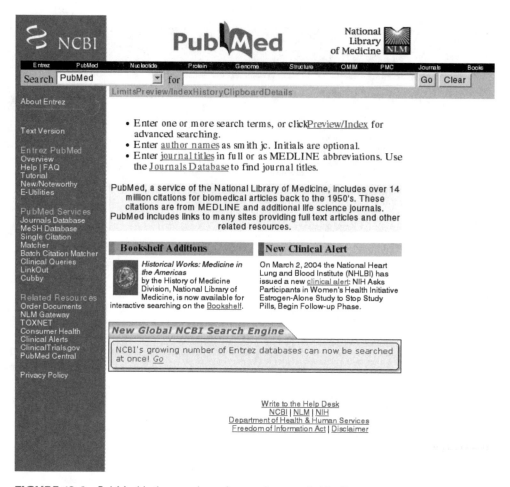

FIGURE 10.4 PubMed is the search engine used to search Medline.

nection with their own physicians. Not only is the information likely to be reliable, but also some found an e-mail consultation less intimidating than a face-to-face meeting, enabling them to ask questions that they would not otherwise ask. Yet, few doctors make it available. Doctors express concerns with the time it would take to read and respond to e-mail, problems of liability, and issues of confidentiality and privacy. However, one 3-year study of a pediatric practice, which offered free e-mail as an option, found it was an effective way for doctors and patients and their families to communicate. In 33 months, a total of 1,239 e-mails were received from parents (81 percent) and health care providers (19 percent) alike. Some requested general information (69 percent); others had specific questions (22 percent). Most (87 percent) were answered immediately with suggested treatment and the recommendation to see a doctor. "On average, reading and responding to each e-mail took slightly less than 4 minutes" (Borowitz, 1998).

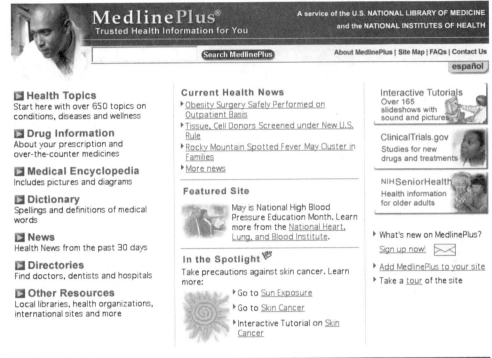

FIGURE 10.5 MEDLINEPlus is a database maintained for consumers.

Other practices do not deal with e-mail in the same way. In a study of unsolicited e-mail, a fictitious patient sent e-mail to 58 dermatology Web sites around the world. Although the message asked for help with a problem that required attention immediately, only one-half the sites responded. However, of those that responded, more than 90 percent recommended that the patient see a doctor; and 59 percent diagnosed the condition correctly. A questionnaire was sent to the sites that had responded. Twenty-eight percent said that they usually do not answer any patient e-mail. Only 24 percent said they answer e-mail communications individually.

In April 2002, a survey was conducted asking doctors and patients for their attitudes towards e-mail. It found that 90 percent of patients would like to exchange e-mail with their physicians, while only 15 percent of doctors do exchange e-mail with their patients. Doctors cite concerns with liability (a paper trail), privacy, time, the possibilities of misunderstanding, and the slowness of e-mail compared with conversation. The small percent of doctors who provide e-mail state that patients are

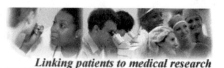

ClinicalTrials.gov

A service of the National Institutes of Health
Developed by the National Library of Medicine

Linking patients to medical research

Home | Search | Browse | Resources | Help | What's New | About

ClinicalTrials.gov provides regularly updated information about federally and privately supported clinical research in human volunteers. ClinicalTrials.gov gives you information about a trial's purpose, who may participate, locations, and phone numbers for more details. Before searching, you may want to learn more about clinical trials.

Search Clinical Trials

Example: heart attack, Los Angeles

[   ]   Search | Tips

Search by Specific Information

Focused Search - search by disease, location, treatment, sponsor...

Browse

Browse by Condition - studies listed by disease or condition
Browse by Sponsor - studies listed by funding organization

Resource Information

Understanding Clinical Trials - information explaining and describing clinical trials
What's New - studies in the news
MedlinePlus - authoritative consumer health information
Genetics Home Reference - consumer information about genes and genetic conditions
NIH Health Information - research supported by the National Institutes of Health

U.S. National Library of Medicine Contact NLM Customer Service
National Institutes of Health, Department of Health & Human Services
Copyright, Privacy, Accessibility, Freedom of Information Act

FIGURE 10.6 ClinicalTrials.gov is a Web site providing information on current clinical trials.

calmer when they know there is an open line to their physicians, and therefore don't need to communicate as much. Some doctors who provide e-mail for their patients maintain "no malpractice lawsuits . . . had been filed in which e-mail played a role" (Hafner, 2002).

Self-help on the Web

Tens of millions of adults search the Web for health-related information. Some people visiting health-related Web sites may just be doing academic research or seeking to learn. However, many are looking for a diagnosis, treatment, and cure. The number of sites either providing advice or linking to sites that provide advice are too numerous to list. Many sites include disclaimers stating in general, that, although they attempt to include only accurate information, they are not responsible for the validity of the information presented. The disclaimer may further advise that a medical professional be consulted before any treatment is either started or discontinued. There are sites devoted to almost any disease, condition, treatment, and drug. You can find self-help for depression, stress, addiction, and almost any personal problem you can name. You do not even need to name your problem. One site shows you a human body and invites you to click where it hurts. You are then presented with a list of possible body parts and their possible diseases. If you continue to click, you will be linked to sites that can provide you with information and advice, from "how to treat your own" to where to go for professional help.

Information is not the only online health-related resource. A possibly dangerous development is the availability of both prescription and nonprescription drugs on the Web. The sale of drugs over the Internet is virtually unregulated. A person can log on in one state, find a pharmacy in another state, "consult" (over telecommunications lines) with a doctor, who will then write a prescription, which will be filled through the mail. The prescriptions are signed by physicians whose "examination" of the "patient" may consist of a review of a short questionnaire. Several states are investigating this development, which is (according to several medical boards) either "illegal or does not meet accepted standards of care." Nonprescription drugs are also available.

Support Groups on the Web

The Web provides online support. There are support groups for hospitalized children, people with cancer and other diseases, and for their families and caregivers. Newsgroups, e-mail discussion groups, and live chat groups are available that link people with health- or disease-related interests. **Starbright World** is a network linking 30,000 seriously ill children in 100 hospitals and many homes in North America. Children in the network can play games, chat, and send and receive e-mail. They can also get medical information.

Support groups exist for virtually every illness. When Dr. Ken Mott, a public health physician, was diagnosed with cancer, he had to travel to receive the treatment he needed. Illness can be isolating. Being in a strange city can compound the isolation. But Dr. Mott, like many other patients, found support and community on the World Wide Web. "Physical disability and pain . . . physical and emotional isolation occur. . . . The . . . side effects of treatment . . . leave victims susceptible to depression and withdrawal. But on the Internet and through e-mail I find dimensions of communication for emotional and psychological support that you may not have imagined." It is especially helpful for people with rare diseases. Takayasu arteritis occurs in between 1.2 to 2.6 people per million scattered over the world, making it virtually impossible to form face-to-face support groups. Yet, now the Internet is being used to build a community and disseminate information and give support.

Judging the Reliability of Health Information on the Internet

Anyone can offer information on the Web, with possibly dangerous results. A compliance officer at the FDA related one instance: "A physician was browsing the Web when he came across a site that contained a fraudulent drug offering. . . . the person who maintains the site claimed he had a cure for a very serious disease, and advised those with the disease to stop taking their prescription medication. Instead they were told to buy the product he was selling, at a cost of several hundred dollars" (Health Information On-Line, 1996). Web sites can be run by anyone. More and more sites providing medical information are being operated by unidentified sources, vendors, and manufacturers; many sites are produced by patients. Judging the reliability of a Web site can be difficult. The U.S. Department of Health and Human Services has established a site to help guide people toward reliable sources of information.

In addition, in response to the need to judge the reliability of health information on the Internet, commercial online services have been created. They will research information and clinical trials for you for a fee of between $150 and $500. There are only 10 small companies, and no one judges their reliability. Users are advised to look into the qualifications of the searchers, and make sure they do not receive any money from drug companies. Of course, users do not have to hire a service to judge information.

The American Medical Association advises users to judge Web sites as critically as they would judge printed information. The number one concern of people using the Web for medical information is privacy. Even though most sites have stated privacy policies, a study found that most do not adhere to them. Users have no way of knowing this. The actual content of the site should be judged on the following criteria: Is there information on the author, and is the author reliable? Are the sources of information clear and reliable? Are the sources of funding revealed? Are there any conflicts of interest, for example, does the author or site receive money from any source interested in steering the user toward a particular treatment? Is the information up-to-date?

Even reliable sites can provide partial information to doctors as well as patients. According to one physician, the Web is as attractive to physicians as it is to patients. But even the best sites are incomplete at best. A MEDLINE search produces abstracts of articles, not the articles themselves. The abstract states the conclusion of a study, for example, that a heart drug was found to be effective, but that is not enough information. The abstract leaves out the necessary details: Who were the participants and how were they selected? What other medications were they taking? How was the data analyzed? Who designed and financed the study?

Reliable sites do exist. The Virtual Hospital is a comprehensive and authoritative site, which has been maintained by the University of Iowa since 1992. It provides information for patients and health care providers. Its information comes from 350 peer-reviewed sources. Every page displayed contains the author's name, degree, and the peer-review status of the content. Material is presented in multimedia format and is organized both by type of information (e.g., textbook) and by problem. A health care provider can read a chapter on upper respiratory conditions and view a video clip of the condition. Providers can also complete continuing education credits through the Virtual Hospital by taking an online test. The Virtual Hospital provides information for patients on disease prevention, including immunizations, diet, and cancer screening. Reliable information is also available through Medscape, which provides a collection of medical journals online.

SELF-HELP SOFTWARE

For those without an Internet connection, self-help software on CD-ROM provides information, suggests diagnoses and treatments, and may even act as a therapist for people with mild to moderate emotional problems, including stress, eating disorders, sexual dysfunction, and depression. Before attempting any self-treatment or taking any medication (even over-the-counter nonprescription medications), before taking advice on the Internet, you should always check with your physician.

Family health guides on CD-ROM provide more information than a book and are easier to search. According to the president of the Consumer Health Information Research Institute, "They cover a lot of general information very well."

The information you need is on your screen at the click of a mouse. The *Mayo Clinic Family Health Book on CD-ROM* is a comprehensive source of information on health, illness, and medication. The user can quickly learn from text, graphics, and video how to stop a bleeding cut. The *Doctor's Book of Home Remedies* is a source of information on alternative remedies—such as garlic and salt water for a cold. *Medical HouseCall* allows the user to enter his or her symptoms and responds with possible diagnoses, as well as advice on calling the doctor. Some programs allow the user to enter complete medical histories for each family member. Other guides focus on medications, or fitness, or a specific condition.

Some psychologists see a place for self-help along with professional therapy. Computers are being used as a tool to screen teenagers for a variety of conditions, including suicidal tendencies. A program developed at Columbia University College of Physicians and Surgeons prompts the interviewer to ask 3,000 questions and follow-ups. Anyone flagged by the computer is seen by a psychologist who then makes the diagnosis. Many psychological diagnostic tests are self-administered. One company advertises self-administered tests that they claim will help diagnose addiction, thought errors, and even criminal tendencies. They do warn, however, that these diagnoses are meant as suggestions only; they are not conclusive.

CONCLUSION

Information technology, specifically the explosive growth of the Internet, has made more information available to more people than ever before. However, the quality of the information varies. Moreover, access is not equally distributed across society, but is restricted to those with computers with Internet connections. Both health care professionals and consumers use these new informational resources. The effects of the use of expert systems and extensive medical literature databases available to health care professionals have not been extensively studied. They apparently do improve physician performance in some areas. There is accurate general information available for health care consumers. However, extreme caution must be exercised in using the Internet or self-help software as a source of health care information.

SELECTED READING

Anahad O'Connor. "Images of Preserved Embryos to Become a Learning Tool." *New York Times,* March 25, 2003.

IN THE NEWS

Images of Preserved Embryos to Become a Learning Tool
by Anahad O'Connor

For 115 years, thousands of embryos that were lost in miscarriages have been preserved for study at the National Museum of Health and Medicine of the Armed Forces Institute of Pathology in Washington.

Now, in an effort to make the embryos, known as the Carnegie Collection, accessible to students and scientists all over the world, scientists at Louisiana State University are translating some of the 7,000 embryos to digital.

The goal of the project, called the Virtual Human Embryo, is to put together thousands of detailed images from the collection on a series of DVDs and CD-ROMs, which can be ordered from the project's Web site, virtualhumanembryo.lsuhsc.edu, at only the cost of shipping and handling.

Human embryo development is divided into 23 stages over eight weeks; after that point, the embryo becomes a fetus with distinguishable human features.

"Essentially, at least one embryo from each of the 23 stages is serially sectioned into multiple slices and a computer captures digital images of each slice under a microscope," said Dr. Raymond F. Gasser, a cell biologist and anatomist at the Louisiana State Health Sciences Center at New Orleans who leads the project.

The images are electronically enhanced and stitched together with corresponding sections to recreate the embryo digitally. Each section is also electronically restained and cleaned up to remove debris, said Dr. Gasser, so that the digital images are in better condition than the original sections in Washington.

Doing this for an embryo from Stage 1, a one-cell zygote, is fairly simple, Dr. Gasser said. But a Stage 23 embryo, which is a little over an inch long, requires roughly 3,000 sections—an arduous task.

The program lets users manipulate colorful three-dimensional reconstructions of the embryos, zoom in and out of the embryonic tissue, and find specific parts of the embryos. Another option lets users "scan," top to bottom, through the embryo.

"Human embryos are small and opaque, which makes them hard to study," said Dr. Gary Schoenwolf, an embryology professor at the University of Utah, who is using the program in his medical school classes. "But this technology acts somewhat like a bologna slicer, letting you create stacks of slices that you can look at in amazing detail or use to recreate and rotate the bologna in three dimensions."

Understanding how an embryo develops, Dr. Schoenwolf added, will better prepare scientists to prevent birth defects.

CHAPTER SUMMARY

This chapter introduced the reader to the vast informational resources made available by computer technology and the Internet.

- Computer-assisted-instruction has been used in the education of health care professionals since the 1960s.
  - Drill-and-practice software teaches facts that require memorization.
  - Simulations teach students to evaluate situations and solve problems, as well as teaching skills. Some simulation programs use data from the Visible Human—an ongoing project that contains thousands of images of one male and one female cadaver.
  - Currently, simulation programs are making use of virtual reality techniques, so that the student actually feels as if he or she were performing a procedure. Simulations using virtual reality are used to teach many skills, including surgical procedures, administration of epidural anesthesia, and dentistry.
  - Patient simulators provide realistic programmable mannequins on which students can practice procedures.
  - Computers and telecommunications have made distance learning possible.
- Expert systems such as INTERNIST, MYCIN, and POEMS are used as decision support systems to help in diagnosis.
- The Internet makes a huge amount of information (and misinformation) available to both health care providers and patients. The effects of its use have not yet been evaluated.
  - Medical literature databases such as MEDLINE provide access to the latest research.
  - The Internet provides opportunities for lifelong, distance learning for health care professionals.

- Health-related information on the Web can be accurate (such as that provided by the Virtual Hospital) or of dubious value. The user must use caution and common sense. The Internet also has online support groups for people with illnesses and for their families.
- Self-help software is available on CD-ROM and, if used with caution, may provide useful information.

KEY TERMS

ADAM
Centerwatch
Clinical Pharmacology
ClinicalTrials.gov
Databank for
    Cardiovascular
    Disease
explorable virtual
    human
ILIAD
INTERNIST
KISMET
MediSpan

MEDLARS (Medical Lit-
    erature Analysis and
    Retrieval System)
MEDLINE
MYCIN
new medicines in
    development
PediaSim
PubMed
PLATO (Programmed
    Logic for Automatic
    Teaching
    Operations)

Post Operative Expert
    Medical System
    (POEMS)
SDILINE (Selective
    Dissemination of
    Information
    onLINE)
Starbright World
virtual hospital
virtual human embryo
Visible Human Project

REVIEW QUESTIONS

Multiple Choice

1. The most comprehensive medical literature database is _____.
   A. SDILINE
   B. AIDSLINE
   C. MEDLINE
   D. None of the above
2. _____ is a programmable mannequin of a child on which students can practice procedures.
   A. Childsim
   B. PediaSim
   C. The Small Virtual Patient
   D. None of the above
3. _____ is an expert system that helps in diagnosis.
   A. MYCIN
   B. INTERNIST
   C. None of the above
   D. A and B are both expert systems

4. _____ is a computerized library of human anatomy.
   A. The Visible Human Project
   B. The Virtual Hospital
   C. The Databank of Cardiovascular Disease
   D. None of the above

5. The best place to look for *authoritative* general health care information online for consumers would be _____.
   A. MEDLINEPlus
   B. Centerwatch
   C. Any search will find authoritative information
   D. There is no reliable information on the Internet.

6. Which of the following is likely to be a source of reliable health care information on the Internet?
   A. A site maintained by a drug company
   B. A site maintained by a patient
   C. A site maintained by a university
   D. None of the above is likely to provide reliable information.

7. _____ is a database of the most recent additions to MEDLINE.
   A. MEDLARS
   B. AIDSLINE
   C. NEWLINE
   D. SDILINE

8. Which of the following is currently being taught with the aid of simulations using virtual reality?
   A. Minimally invasive surgical techniques
   B. The administration of epidural anesthesia
   C. Some aspects of dentistry
   D. All of the above

9. _____ is a program that teaches anatomy by allowing the student to use a mouse to click away layers of the body.
   A. ILIAD
   B. ADAM
   C. KISMET
   D. None of the above

10. It is not difficult to find support groups on the Web. Starbright World _____.
    A. attempts to link seriously ill children in hospitals in the United States
    B. Is a network of AIDS patients
    C. Is a network of people with cancer
    D. Is a network of families of people with cancer

True/False Questions

1. Expert systems will eventually replace doctors. _____
2. All the information on the Internet is reliable and accurate. _____
3. MEDLARS is a collection of medical literature databases. _____

4. The Visible Human Project provides anatomically detailed, three-dimensional representations of the male and female human body. _____
5. The Virtual Hospital is a service of the University of Iowa that provides up-to-date, accurate health-related information on the Web. _____
6. In order to post health-related information on the Internet, a person needs to pass a rigorous exam. _____
7. Information on current clinical drug trials is available on the Internet. _____
8. Some studies have contended that there are programs that may be helpful in treating mild clinical depression. _____
9. ADAM is a program that teaches anatomy. _____
10. Simulation programs began to be used in health care education in the 1990s. _____

Critical Thinking

1. Discuss the advantages and disadvantages of using virtual reality simulations in health care education.
2. It is possible to become a physician assistant in a distance learning program without being physically present on a campus or setting foot in a classroom. How do you think this might affect education?
3. Given the many uses of information technology in health care today, anyone entering a health care field must be computer literate and computer competent. Discuss this statement.
4. The Internet provides unparalleled informational resources for both consumers and providers of health care. This may be helpful. However, it may be quite dangerous. Comment on the positive and negative aspects of the availability of health-related information on the Internet.
5. One of the characteristics of the Internet is anonymity—you can hide our identity, and so can anyone else. Discuss the possible effects of this on Internet support groups.

SOURCES

ADAM. http://www.adam.com (2003; October 26, 2003).
Aschoff, Susan. "A Diehard Patient." sptimes.com (April 30, 2002; September 10, 2003).
Association of Schools of Public Health Distance Programs. asph.org (2003; October 26, 2003).
Beamish, Rita. "Computers Now Helping to Screen for Troubled Teen-Agers." *New York Times,* December 17, 1998, p. G9.
Bitzer, Maryann D., and Martha C. Boudreaux. "Using a Computer to Teach Nursing," reprinted from *Nursing Forum,* 1969. In *Computers in Nursing,* ed. Rita D. Zielstorff. Rockville, MD: Aspen, 1982, pp. 171–85.
Borowitz, Stephen, and Jeffrey Wyatt. "The Origin, Content, and Workload of E-mail Consultations" (Abstract). *JAMA* (October 21, 1998): 1360–61.
CIDI Composite International Diagnostic Interview. http://www.who.int/msa/cidi/index-orig.htm (1999; October 13, 2003).
CIDI Literature Review. http://www.who.int/msa/cidi/literature.htm (October 16, 1998; October 13, 2003).

Classen, D. C. "Clinical Decision Support Systems to Improve Clinical Practice and Quality of Care," Editorial. *JAMA* (October 21, 1998): 1360–61.

"Considerations for the Use of E-mail and the Internet by Physicians and Patients." http://www.ama-assn.org/sci-pubs/sci-news/1998/snr1021.htm#/joc80319 (October 21, 1998; October 26, 2003).

Digital Divide. geocities.com/tcanada1301/divide.html (2002; September 13, 2003).

A DOD SBIR Success Story. http://www.dodsbir.com/materials/SuccessStories/ImmersionMedical.htm (n.d.; October 12, 2003).

Dorsey, Coston et al. "Emergency Room Triage System." vt.edu/business/sumichrast/5474F96/ER_Sm96.pdf (1996; October 26, 2003).

Eisenberg, Anne. "The Virtual Stomach (No, It's Not a Diet Aid)." nyt.com (October 31, 2002; November 1, 2002).

Eng, Thomas R., Andrew Maxfield, Kevin Patrick, Mary J. Deering, Scott C. Ratzan, and David H. Gustafson. "Access to Health Information and Support: A Public Highway or a Private Road?" (Abstract). *JAMA* (October 21, 1998): 1371–75.

Epstein, Randi Hutter. "Sifting through the Online Medical Jumble." nyt.com (January 28, 2003; January 30, 2003).

"Evaluating Medical Information on the Internet." AARP. www.aarp.org/health (March 17, 2003; September 17, 2003).

Expert Trainer. hmc.psu.edu (September 9, 2003; October 12, 2003).

Fact Sheet. "The Visible Human Project." nlm.nih.gov (February 16, 2001; September 12, 2003).

Ferguson, Tom. "Digital Doctoring—Opportunities and Challenges in Electronic Patient-Physician Communication," Editorial. *JAMA* (October 21, 1998): 1361–62.

Fisk, Sandra. "Doc in a Box: A Home Health Software Guide." *Better Homes and Gardens* (August 1995): 44–52.

Griffin, Susan. "Virtual Dentistry Becomes Reality in Multimedia Labs." http://www.cwru.edu/pubs/cnews/2001/9-27/dent-sim.htm (2001; October 13, 2003).

Guernsey, Lisa. "A Dissent on the Digital Divide." nyt.com (September 18, 2003; September 20, 2003).

Hafner, Katie. "Why Doctors Don't E-mail." nyt.com (June 6, 2002; August 30, 2002).

Hamilton, Robert A. "FDA Examining Computer Diagnosis." *FDA Consumer Magazine* (September 1995). http://www.fda.gov/fdac/features/795_compdiag.html (September 1995; June 10, 1999).

"Health Information On-line." *FDA Consumer,* June 1996, revised Jan. 1998, http://www.fda.gov/fdac/features/596_info.html (January 1998; June 10, 1999).

Hersh, William, and David Hickam. "How Well Do Physicians Use Electronic Information Retrieval Systems? A Framework for Investigation and Systematic Review" (Abstracts). *JAMA* (October 21, 1998): 1347–52.

"How to Evaluate Health Information on the Internet: Questions and Answers." cis.nci.nih.gov (August 28, 2002; September 17, 2003).

"KISMET 3-D Simulation Software: A 'Virtual Reality' Based Training System for Minimally Invasive Surgery." http://ireg1.iai.fzk.de/TRAINER/mic_trainer1.html, (July 10, 2001; September 13, 2003).

Kolata, Gina. "Web Research Transforms Visit to the Doctor." nyt.com (March 6, 2000; March 6, 2000).

Le, Tao. "Medical Education and the Internet: This Changes Everything." *JAMA* 285, no. 6 (February 14, 2001): 809.

Lindberg, Donald A. B. "The National Library of Medicine's Web Site for Physicians and Patients." MS *JAMA* 285, no. 6 (February 14, 2001): 806.

Maddox, Peggy Jo. "Ethics and the Brave New World of E-Health."
    http://www.nursingworld.org (November 21, 2002; March 18, 2003).
"Medical Databases." medic8.com (2003; October 26, 2003).
"Medical Databases." allhealthnet.com (March 19, 2002; October 26, 2003).
Mott, Ken. "Cancer and the Internet." *Newsweek,* August 19, 1996, p. 19.
National Library of Medicine's Visible Human Project.
    http://www.nlm.nih.gov/research/visible/visible_human.html (September 11, 2003;
    October 26, 2003).
O'Connor, Anahad. "Images of Preserved Embryos to Become a Learning Tool," nyt.com
    (March 25, 2003; March 26, 2003).
Patient Simulator Program, HPS Capabilities. cscc.edu (n.d.; September 5, 2003).
Patsos, Mary. "The Internet and Medicine: Building a Community for Patients with Rare
    Diseases." *JAMA* 285 no. 6 (February 14, 2001): 805.
PediaSim Capabilities. Cscc.edu (2000; September 5, 2003).
Prutkin, Jordan. "Cybermedical Skills for the Internet Age." *JAMA* 285, no. 6 (February 14,
    2001): 808.
Psych Screen, Inc. psychscreen.com (n.d.; September 12, 2003).
"Public Health Workforce Development." phf.org (May 12, 2003; October 26, 2003).
Rajendran, Pam R. "The Internet: Ushering in a New Era of Medicine." *JAMA* 285, no. 6
    (February 14, 2001): 804–5.
Rubin, Rita. "Prescribing on Line . . . Industry's Rapid Growth, Change Defy Regulation."
    USA Today, October 2, 1998, pp. 1, 2.
"Safety Data from FDA." *New York Times,* (October 10, 1998), p. G10.
Speilberg, Alissa. "On Call and Online, Sociohistorical, Legal and Ethical Implications of
    E-mail for the Patient-Physician Relationship" Abstracts. *JAMA* (October 21, 1998):
    1353–59.
Starbright World. starbright.org (n.d.; September 12, 2003).
Terry, Nicolas. "Access vs. Quality Assurance: The E-Health Conundrum." *JAMA* 285, no. 6
    (February 14, 2001): 807.
"Tour of the Virtual Hospital, A" vh.org/welcome/tour (2003; October 26, 2003).
Trowbridge, Robert, and Scott Weingarten. *Making Health Care Safer: A Critical Analysis of
    Patient Safety Practices.* Evidence Report/Technology Assessment: Number 43. AHRQ
    Publication No. 01-E058, July 2001. Agency for Healthcare Research and Quality,
    Rockville, MD. http://www.ahrq.gov/clinic/ptsafety/ Clinical Decision Support
    Systems.
"2001 Report to Congress on Telemedicine, Telehealth." hrsa.gov/pubs/report2001 (May 16,
    2002; October 9, 2003).
Udeshi, Ashish. "VR meets OR." digital.library.Miami.edu (n.d., but after 2002; October 27,
    2003).
Urbankova, Alice, and Richard Lichtenthal. "DentSim Virtual Reality in Preclinical
    Operative Dentistry to Improve Psychomotor Skills: A Pilot Study." denx.com. (2002;
    October 26, 2003).
Virtual Hospital. vh.org (n.d.; September 12, 2003).
Versweyveld, Leslie. "KISMET Simulation Software Forms Heart of the Karlsruhe
    Endoscopic Surgery Trainer." http://www.hoise.com/vmw/articles/LV-VM-09-08-
    10.html (July 6, 1998; May 13, 2004).
Visible Human Project. nlm.nih.gov (September 11, 2003; May 13, 2004).
Visible Human Project: From Data to Knowledge, The. nlm.nih.gov/research/visible/
    data2knowledge.html (May 3, 2001; September 10, 2003).

"Web of Wealth." *USA Today,* November 2, 1998, p. D1.

"What's New in the Virtual Hospital?" vh.org (n.d.; September 12, 2003).

Wilson, Dick. "Virtual Reality Takes the Risk Out of Training." CNN Interactive, Sci-Tech. http://www.nlm.nih.gov/research/visible/visible_human.html October 2, 1997.

Winker, Margaret A., Annette Flanagin, Bonnie Chi-Lum, John White, Karen Andrews, Robert L. Kennett, Catherine D. DeAngelis, and Robert A. Musacchio. "Guidelines for Medical and Health Information on the Internet." journals.iranscience.net:800/ ama-assn.org (August 7, 2001; October 26, 2003).

Zuger, Abigail. "Reams of Information, Some of It Even Useful." nyt.com (October 25, 2000; October 26, 2003).

RELATED WEB SITES

The Federal Trade Commission (FTC) looks into complaints about false health claims on the Internet. Their Web page can help consumers evaluate claims.

http://www.ftc.gov/bcp/conline/edcams/cureall is the Federal Trade Commission's *Operation Cure-all* page.

The Food and Drug Administration (FDA) regulates drugs and medical devices. *Buying Medicines and Medical Products Online* is at http:///www.fda.gov/oc/buyonline.

The National Cancer Institute is located at http://cancer.gov.

The Harvard School of Public Health provides consumers with *Ten Questions to Help Make Sense of Health Headlines* at www.health-insight.com.

The *Journal of the American Medical Association* is available at jama.ama-assn.org.

The National Library of Medicine provides access to Medline and MEDLINEPlus at www.nlm.nih.gov.

Conclusion and Future Directions

OUTLINE

- **Learning Objectives**
- **Overview**
- **Clinical and Special Purpose Applications: Future Trends**
- **Administrative Applications: The Integrated Electronic Medical Record**
- **Demographic Changes and Occupational Outlooks for Health Care Professionals**
- **Social Implications**
- **Chapter Summary**
- **Sources**

LEARNING OBJECTIVES

Chapter 11 summarizes developments in information technology as they relate to health care. Upon completion of this chapter, you will be able to

- Summarize new developments in clinical and special purpose applications of IT to health care.
- Discuss new administrative applications, specifically the use of the electronic medical record.
  - List the advantages and disadvantages associated with the use of the electronic medical record.
- Describe demographic changes and their impact on occupational outlook for health care professionals.
- Describe the social implications of the applications of information technology to health care.

OVERVIEW

Information technology has transformed many aspects of our society, including health care. Over the past quarter century the development of clinical and special purpose applications has contributed to more accurate and less invasive methods of diagnosis and treatment. The ability to deliver health care services via telecommunications lines can potentially transform the distribution of health services, making the human and technical resources of major medical centers available wherever there is a computer with a broadband connection to the Internet.

The use of computers in health care administration continues to expand. Although the first use of computer technology in health care was in administrative areas, the electronic medical record, which would integrate all patient information, has not yet been universally adopted. With the spread of managed care, however, the computerization of patient information has accelerated.

CLINICAL AND SPECIAL PURPOSE APPLICATIONS: FUTURE TRENDS

Some areas of health care, such as radiology, surgery, and pharmacy, are in the process of being transformed by computer technology. CT scans, MRIs, and PET scans use digital imaging techniques to create highly detailed and accurate images of the structure and function of the human body. The precision of these images has decreased the need for exploratory surgery, thus reducing pain and the costs of hospitalization. These images can help guide surgery when it is necessary. The replacement of the traditional X-ray on film by the digital X-ray, which can be viewed on a monitor, makes it possible to focus on particular problem areas and to share images. Interventional radiologists using radiosurgery and focused ultrasound can now treat conditions that once required traditional surgery. Still newer tools are being developed. New photography hardware and software for finding early signs of melanoma are being used at Duke University. Photographs are digitized and transferred to CD-ROM. The images are shown on a monitor. Any suspicious area can then be more closely examined on the screen. Now not even the brain is a mystery; its functioning can be studied using PET scans and functional MRIs.

Computers have become a necessary component in surgery, from the teaching and planning stages where simulations can be used, to the actual operating room where a surgeon may be assisted by AESOP holding a laparoscope. Computers have also spurred the development of minimally invasive surgical techniques, which lead to less scarring and pain, and lower costs. Systems that allow the remote operation of a scalpel have been developed to cushion the vibrations of a surgeon's hands. Telepresence or distance surgeries have been successfully performed with many miles separating the surgeon and patient.

New computer-based techniques are being used in the dentist's office. From the use of an electronic appointment book and medical record to the diagnosing and filling of cavities, information technology has found its place in dentistry. New techniques using light are being utilized to find cavities too small for examinations or X-rays to see. Lasers of different lengths can be used to sculpt the gum or drill a cavity.

In pharmacy, robots are taking the place of human beings in filling prescriptions in both hospital and community pharmacies. Computers help in several ways in the development of new drugs. The Human Genome Project, made possible by the capacity of computers to store, organize, and make accessible vast amounts of data instantly, is providing us with a clearer understanding of human genetics and, therefore, the genetic bases of some diseases. Knowledge of the molecular basis of a disease can lead to better prediction, prevention, and improvements in diagnosis and treatment. It has led to the development of several drugs in the last few years. In the future, a fuller appreciation of the human genome may make it possible to actually grow replacement body parts or stimulate the body to repair itself! The Physiome Project promises the development of models of organs and of a whole virtual patient on which to experiment with drugs and treatments before actual clinical trials are started.

The microprocessor has improved medical devices of all kinds. Medical instruments with embedded microprocessors are more accurate than their predecessors. Adaptive devices help those with impaired vision, speech, hearing, and mobility to live independent, productive lives. Computerized prosthetics may work as well as natural limbs. FES technology can keep paralyzed muscles from becoming atrophied, and can even restore movement. What was impossible yesterday is now possible. Some examples are a blind person seeing, someone paralyzed by a spinal injury being able to walk, a stroke victim being able to communicate via thoughts magnified by a microchip implanted in his or her brain, or the speech of a mute stroke victim being restored by an implanted microchip. Work is now underway on brain-computer interfaces, so that surgery will not be necessary.

New devices emerge every day from pacemakers that can communicate over the Internet to the experimental VeriChip, which may in the future be implanted and linked to a database of medical information. Other devices that depend on microprocessors and sophisticated software are also in development: a toothbrush that checks for bacteria and blood sugar and sends the information to your medical record; glasses that help with memory; skin surface mapping that detects melanoma early; smart bandages that can detect bacteria and viruses and inform the wearer if an antibiotic is needed; a wheelchair, controlled by voice or a touch pad that finds its own way through a crowded room or subway platform. A brain prosthetic—a chip that mimics the hippocampus (responsible for memory)—is in the very early stages of development. Other implants in development can help grow bones. In October 2003, scientists reported that "a monkey with electrodes implanted in its brain could move a robot arm, much as if it were moving its own arm" (Blakeslee 2003). Doctors and scientists are continuing the research, attempting to adapt the device for paralyzed patients. In the future, nanotechnology may diagnose and treat disease at the molecular level.

Electronic glasses are in the development stage. These smart glasses will be able to automatically focus and refocus. Traditional glasses bend light with their lens shape. Electronic glasses will contain software, chips, and material sensitive to the application of electrical voltage. The latter will change the refraction of the material in the lens. Each pixel in the lens can have different amounts of electricity applied. Problems have to be solved before these glasses are ready to be sold to the public. Glasses have to transmit light. However, currently these glasses absorb light.

Not only have traditional areas of health care been transformed, but also whole new fields, such as telemedicine, have emerged, and continue to expand at a rapid rate. The delivery of health care over telecommunications lines includes the sharing of images and records, distance consultations and exams, and the remote operation of medical equipment. It is now being used to deliver health care in some rural areas, to day care centers, to isolated stroke patients, to prisoners, and to the homebound elderly. If the necessary broadband lines are put into place, telemedicine can expand to bring the most current knowledge and expertise anywhere that there is a computer and a broadband link to the Internet. Telepharmacy is expanding due to U.S. federal government interest, and telesurgery is receiving funding from the Canadian federal government. Telehome care is seen as a way to cut costs while improving care. The sale of home-care devices is growing at a rapid pace.

Computer technology has changed the way we teach and learn. Computer-assisted instruction includes both drill-and-practice and simulation software. Virtual reality simulations help teach a variety of skills to health care providers. Simulated patients allow students to practice procedures under close to real conditions. Databases of medical information make the latest research available anywhere there is a computer with an Internet connection. Expert systems can be used successfully as an aid in diagnosis. Medical information (of vastly differing quality) is available on the Internet and the World Wide Web to more and more people—allowing health care consumers and providers to educate themselves, patients to find support groups, and professionals to communicate with colleagues and patients.

New sites have emerged that judge the quality of other sites, and organizations like the American Medical Association have published guidelines of what consumers should look for in judging a medical Web site.

ADMINISTRATIVE APPLICATIONS: THE INTEGRATED ELECTRONIC MEDICAL RECORD

The earliest use of computers in health care was in administration. Hospitals instituted computerized budgeting and financial planning; medical offices used programs specifically designed for their needs. However, standardization of record keeping and the integration of computer systems via the complete electronic medical patient record lagged. Something as simple as introducing a standardized computerized sign-out system that lists patients' problems, treatments, and medications, so that incoming staff are fully informed, was found in a recent study to improve patient care. There is no way to tell the extent of the adoption of the electronic medical record. Probably most large institutions use a combination of paper charts and electronic records. According to a report published in August 2000, "no more than one family physician in 20 ha[d] adopted the technology" (Lippmann, 2000). Small practices point to the high cost, the huge job of entering data, the difficulty of using many programs, and the fact that the programs do not fit the way these practices work.

HIPAA encourages the use of the EMR, requires new security measures, and is the first law to put a national floor under the privacy of medical information. However, the USA Patriot Act may counteract the increased protection. The adoption of the electronic medical record may be accelerating. A standardized electronic record is peculiarly suited to today's health care system, where medical practices are accountable to outside agencies—whether insurance companies, government agencies, or the HMO business administrator—that measure their performance using business criteria and tend to look first at patient charts.

Ideally, the fully computerized integrated medical record would be a completely clear and legible record (unlike the paper chart). This record would contain a patient's full medical history, including diagnoses, treatments, hospital and doctor visits, prescriptions, allergies, dietary notes, doctor's notes, lists of problems, lab results, health maintenance reminders, and radiology reports. The record would be instantly available to any authorized person. It would be complete, because, on a standardized form, any omissions stand out. Patient information forms could either be read from beginning to end or searched for specific details. Blood levels could be graphed, changes over time seen instantly. Ideally, the computer could catch any human errors, and alert doctors to dangers of allergic reactions or drug interactions. In one study, one automated hospital information system called the HELP system found 60 times the number of adverse drug events as the traditional method. In an Indiana University study, computer-generated reminders to physicians to give flu vaccines to at-risk patients are credited with decreasing hospitalization, Emergency Room visits, and tests for respiratory conditions by 10 to 30 percent. Health maintenance reminders may become a part of the electronic medical record. However, in a small study of these reminders published in 2003, it was found that although 79 percent thought the reminders a good idea, 75 percent of health care providers said that they did not look at health maintenance reminders (blinking icons) on electronic medical records. Almost 63 percent either ignored or forgot the reminders. Only 20 percent said they discussed the reminders with patients (Schellhase, 2003).

With all of a patient's information available, the computer can detect the possibly dangerous interaction of an underlying medical condition with a drug prescribed by any of the patient's health care providers—from the dentist to the therapist to the surgeon. Programs can point to doctors who order what are deemed unnecessary, expensive tests. Before a test is ordered, the computer can display the results of previous tests and prices of the test considered by the physician. One study found that doctors treating outpatients ordered 14 percent fewer tests per visit when using a computer, which may not be a good thing for patients.

With the fragmentation of care fostered by increased specialization and managed care, patients see less of one practitioner and more of a variety of specialists. The electronic medical record makes the patient's complete history and condition available to each doctor, helping to ensure continuity of care. Some doctors who use the electronic medical record find it less time-consuming to fill out than a paper chart.

The problems raised by the electronic medical record include the cost of instituting and maintaining a computerized system, which can be prohibitively high for a small practice, problems of reliability, and problems of security and privacy, which have not been solved. The cost depends on the system installed and can run from $10,000 to well over $1 million. Annual updates are an additional cost. However, doctors who have installed computerized systems maintain that it is cost saving, because it saves on transcription costs and ensures that a patient is billed for every service rendered. A small survey of health care providers published in 2003 found generally positive attitudes toward the EMR (74 percent liked or loved it), although a majority (79 percent) thought they were less productive using the EMR. Seventy-nine percent thought the EMR to be of higher quality than the traditional paper record (Schellhase, 2003). EMRs are only as reliable as the computer network they are on. The network not only needs to be secure from unauthorized users, but also from natural disasters, and power outages of any kind.

Security of records on a network cannot be guaranteed, nor can the identity of the person signing notes or a prescription. It is easier to forge a signature on a computer than on a paper record. Organizations try to deal with this problem by using secret logins to serve as signatures. The methods of keeping unauthorized users from medical records are far from 100 percent guaranteed. Moreover, under managed care, many organizations (from insurance companies to government agencies) and many employees of these organizations are *authorized* to see a record. How does an organization guard against misuse by authorized personnel? There can be training for personnel and there are laws and internal codes of conduct, but this might not be sufficient.

The use of the electronic medical record raises other questions. Is the EMR any real improvement if it is not universally used? That is, if your dentist doesn't use it, those treatments and conditions are not on the record. If it is decided that sensitive information (therapist's records or certain conditions) will not be safe in electronic form, your record is incomplete. Wouldn't it then be just an electronic form of the fragmented paper records that exist now—just less reliable in a power outage and less secure against invasions of privacy? If practitioners assume that the electronic medical record is complete, but it is not, can it cause more problems than it solves?

DEMOGRAPHIC CHANGES AND OCCUPATIONAL OUTLOOKS FOR HEALTH CARE PROFESSIONALS

Demographic changes and changes in the organization of the delivery of health care are combining to improve the occupational outlook for health care professionals. According to the U.S. Bureau of Labor Statistics (BLS), there will be more than 3 million new jobs in health care—"the largest numerical increase of any industry from 1996–2006." The "[e]mployment of registered nurses is expected to grow faster than the average for all occupations through the year 2006." In a later report, the BLS predicted, "About 13 percent of all wage and salary jobs created between 2000 and 2010 will be in health services." Most of the increase will not be in hospitals, but in other settings. Because of the increasing percentage of older people in our population, many health care professionals will work in home health care, assisted living facilities, and in nursing homes. The expansion of opportunities is also related to the fact that more conditions are treatable. Moreover, there is financial pressure on hospitals to release patients as soon as possible and to perform medical services on an outpatient basis. This increases the need for nurses specializing in home health care. Many of the procedures that once were done in hospitals are now done in HMOs and surgicenters, increasing the opportunities for nurses and other health care professionals in such settings. The rapid development of telemedicine is putting some nurses in autonomous positions supervising projects.

SOCIAL IMPLICATIONS

The social organization of health care and its delivery is not a technical issue. Technological developments (accurate CT scans, PET scans, microprocessors embedded in prosthetic limbs, etc.) make more effective health care a possibility; however, they do not make it a reality. The prices of the new technology (e.g., $25,000 for a wheelchair that climbs stairs) put it out of reach of the vast majority of people. Today fewer people have jobs that offer health insurance. In HMOs, medical decisions may be made on business, not medical, grounds. Furthermore, treatments and devices judged experimental are not covered. The continued development of expensive state-of-the-art equipment may complement the current spate of hospital mergers and the centralization of health care organizations. On the other hand, some developments like telemedicine make the use of this equipment (if insurance companies will cover it) available to more people in more places than ever before. Moreover, medical information is available via the Internet—but only to those with a computer and an Internet connection—accentuating social and economic differences. The same can be said of the incredible prosthetic devices becoming available to those with the money or insurance to pay for them.

The application of computer technology to health care and its delivery holds the promise of improving human existence; the benefits are beyond dispute. However, there are problems that must be addressed before the full potential can be realized. Problems of the privacy and security of the medical record, and the increasing importance of financial motives that HMOs bring, were not created by computers, but information technology does exacerbate them. In the end, the technology itself, although it holds the possibility for improving human existence, is not an independent force. Before the promise of the new technology can be realized, questions of privacy and of the ethical and equitable distribution of health care must be addressed.

CHAPTER SUMMARY

This chapter summarized the applications of information technology in health care.

- Clinical and special purpose applications of computer technology continue to change health care.
  - The fields of radiology, surgery, and pharmacy have been transformed by digital technology.
  - The use of microprocessors in medical devices has made monitors more accurate and prosthetics more lifelike. Adaptive technology has made it possible for people with disabilities to live more productive, independent lives.

Implanted microchips may allow the blind to see, the mute to speak. FES allows some paraplegics to walk.
- New fields, such as telemedicine, have come into being and continue to grow. Telepharmacy and telesurgery are expanding due to government investment.
- Dentistry is becoming more and more dependent on computer technology.
- Computers are used in medical education, from drill-and-practice, to complex virtual reality simulations to programmable mannequins. The Internet and World Wide Web have made health care information available to both providers and consumers.
- Administrative applications continue to expand.
  - The use of computers for financial planning, budgeting, billing, and office administration is well established.
  - The use of the electronic medical record is increasing, but is not universal. It raises problems of security, privacy, and reliability. New laws, including HIPAA and the USA Patriot Act, are further affecting the privacy of health information.
- Demographic changes have improved the occupational outlook for health care professionals.
- Technological improvements hold great promise for improving human existence. However, they do not address the issue of the equitable distribution of health care.

SOURCES

Agency for Health Care Policy and Research, Department of Health and Human Services. "Research in Action: Using Computers to Advance Health Care." http://www.ahcpr.gov/research/computer.htm (January 1996; October 26, 2003).

Arent Fox. "State Activity." http://www.arentfox.com (June 6, 1999; October 26, 2003).

Blakeslee, Sandra. "Imagining Thought-Controlled Movement for Humans." nyt.com (October 14, 2003; October 15, 2003).

Bluth, Andrew. "Wire It, and They Will Come." *New York Times,* December 24, 1998, pp. G1, G8.

Bureau of Labor Statistics. *1998–99 Occupational Outlook Handbook.* http://stats/bls.gov/oco/ocos083.htm (February 26, 1999; June 6, 1999).

Bureau of Labor Statistics. *2002–2003 Occupational Outlook Handbook.* www.bls.gov (2003; October 12, 2003).

Cooke, Darren. "Attitudes about Electronic Medical Record Keeping." Updated 12/4/95. http://www.med.ufl.edu/medinfo /smic95/abs03.html (December 4, 1995; October 26, 2003).

Eisenberg, Anne. "What's Next: A Chip That Mimics Neurons, Firing Up the Memory." nyt.com (June 20, 2002; October 11, 2003).

———. "What's Next: Glasses So Smart They Know What You're Looking At." nyt.com (June 28, 2001; August 30, 2002).

———. "Using Computers to Zoom in on Skin Cancer." *New York Times,* December 15, 1998, p. F8.

Electronic Privacy Information Center. "Medical Record Privacy." http://www.epic.org/privacy/medical (March 28, 2002; May 14, 2003).

Federal Telemedicine Legislation 105th Congress, Arent Fox. http://www.crecre.com (n.d.; October 9, 2003).

Federal Telemedicine Update, Federal Telemedicine News. Telemedicine.com (January 22, 2002; October 13, 2003).

Federal Telemedicine Update, Federal Telemedicine News. Telemedicine.com (August 15, 2002; May 27, 2003).

Federal Telemedicine Update, Federal Telemedicine News. Telemedicine.com (August 19, 2002; October 13, 2003).

"Final Modifications to the HIPAA Privacy Regulations." http://www.hallrender.com/pdf000551HA.pdf (2002; March 27, 2003).

Frame, Paul S. "Automated Health Maintenance Reminders: Tools Do Not Make a System" (Editorial). *Journal of the American Board of Family Practice.* jabfp.org (2003; October 27, 2003).

Junnarkar, Sandeep. "Cases: When Rules for Better Care Exact Their Own Cost." *New York Times,* January 5, 1999, p. F6.

Lewis, Carol. "Emerging Trends in Medical Device Technology: Home Is Where the Heart Monitor Is." *FDA Consumer Magazine,* FDA.gov (May–June 2001; May 17, 2003).

Lippmann, Helen. "Making the Move to Electronic Records." *Hippocrates* 14 no. 8. hippocrates.com (August 2000; October 27, 2003).

Medical Privacy. epic.org (July 6, 2002; October 14, 2003).

O'Mahony, Brian. "The Electronic Medical Record and the Internet." *Journal of Informatics in Primary Care,* (May 1998): 7–11. primis.nhs/informatics/may98/may4.htm (May 1998; October 27, 2003).

Schellhase, Kenneth G., Thomas D. Koepsell, and Thomas E. Norris. "Providers' Reactions to an Automated Health Maintenance Reminder System Incorporated into the Patient's Electronic Medical Record." *Journal of the American Board of Family Practice.* jabfp.org (2003; October 27, 2003).

Stein, Lincoln. "The Electronic Medical Record: Promises and Threats." *Web Journal* 2, no. 3. Web Security: A Matter of Trust. http://www.oreilly.com/catalog/wjsum97/excerpt (1997; October 27, 2003).

Szolovits, Peter. "A Revolution in Electronic Medical Record Systems via the World Wide Web." An extended abstract prepared for a talk at the conference. *The Use of the Internet and World-Wide Web for Telematics in Healthcare.* http://www.medg.1cs.mit.edu/ftp.psz/IAHIT.html (September 1995; October 14, 2003).

2001 Report to Congress on Telemedicine. Telehealth. hrsa.gov/pubs/report2001 (May 16, 2002; October 9, 2003).

Wachter, Glenn. "Telemedicine Legislative Issue Summary." telemed.org (May 2002; March 8, 2003).

Wade, Nicholas. "Blueprints for People, but How to Read Them?" *New York Times,* December 8, 1998, pp. F1, F4.

Wilson, Jennifer Fisher. "How Benefits Can Outweigh Costs of Electronic Records" from *ACP Observer* (April 1998). http://www.acponline.org/journals/news/apr98/ercosts.htm (April 1998; October 27, 2003).

Glossary

ADAM—simulation software that teaches anatomy and physiology, using two- and three-dimensional images (some of them created from the Visible Human data); versions available for both patients and professionals; interactive, allowing the user to click away over 100 layers of the body and see more than 4,000 structures

adaptive technology (assistive technology)—makes it possible for people with disabilities to exercise control over their home and work environments

administrative application—use of information technology for tasks such as office management, finance and accounting, and materials management

AESOP (Automated Endoscopic System for Optimal Positioning)—introduced in 1994 by Computer Motion, Inc., is the first FDA-cleared surgical robot; originally developed for the space program, AESOP is now used as an assistant in endoscopic procedures

Ambulatory patient classification (APC)—reimbursement for hospital outpatient services are based on Ambulatory Patient Classification (APC)

Americans With Disabilities Act of 1990—"federal law which prohibits discrimination against people with disabilities and requires that businesses with more than fifteen employees provide 'reasonable accommodation' to allow the disabled to perform their jobs"

analog device—a device that computes by measuring a physical property; for example, with a mercury thermometer, the length of the column of mercury is measured and is analogous to a number of degrees of temperature

analog signal—a continuous varying wave; traditional telephone lines carry analog waves

antisense technology—one experimental technology used to develop drugs to shut off disease-causing genes; it has not been very successful

APC (ambulatory patient classification)—reimbursement for hospital outpatient services are based on Ambulatory Patient Classification (APC)

application software—programs that perform specific tasks for the user, also called productivity software; include word processing, spreadsheet, database management, graphics, and communications programs.

arithmetic-logic unit—the part of the central processing unit that does arithmetic and logical operations

ARPAnet—a project of the Advanced Research Projects Agency of the U.S. Department of Defense (1969); an attempt to create both a national network of scientists and a communications system that could withstand nuclear attack; later became the Internet

arrhythmia monitor—a device which monitors heart rate

ARTEMIS—a robotic system that works with the simulation software KISMET; allows a surgeon to perform minimally invasive surgery while viewing three screens that show the view presented by the endoscope and simulations

artificial intelligence (AI)—the branch of computer science which seeks to make computers simulate human intelligence

assistive technology—adaptive technology

augmentative communication device—a device that helps those who cannot speak or whose speech is incomprehensible to communicate

augmented reality surgery (enhanced reality surgery)—makes use of computer-generated imagery to provide the surgeon with information that would otherwise be unavailable; these images may either be fused with the image on the monitor or projected directly onto the patient's body during the operation allowing the doctor to virtually see inside the patient

automatic recalculation—refers to the fact that when one value in a spreadsheet is changed, any cell that refers to it is automatically changed

Baby CareLink—a program that links high-risk newborns to their families via telecommunications when the baby is in the hospital and for 6 months after the baby is home; found to shorten hospital stays and give comfort to parents who can see their infants even when they cannot be present at the hospital and can see hospital personnel even when they and their infants are home

bandwidth—a measure of the capacity of transmission media to carry data; the broader the bandwidth, the faster the medium

binary digit (bit)—a one or a zero; binary digits are used to represent data and information in the computer

bioinformatics—the application of information technology to biology

biometric keyboard—a keyboard which can identify a typist by fingerprints

biometric methods—ways of identifying a user by some physical characteristic; include fingerprints, hand prints, retina or iris scans,

lip prints, facial thermography, and body odor sensors

biometrics—the science that measures body characteristics; enables security devices to identify a user by these characteristics

biomicroscopes—tools used for diagnosis of cataracts

biotechnology—discipline which sees the human body as a collection of molecules, and seeks to understand and treat disease in terms of these molecules

bits per second (bps)—a measure of speed in telecommunications

Bluetooth technology—a wireless technology used to link computerized devices, such as a cell phone and pacemaker

body odor sensor—a biometric device enabling the identification of user by odor

boot—load the operating system into memory

cable modem—a modem that connects a computer to a cable TV system that offers online services

CD (compact disk)—optical disk on which data is stored using a laser which burns pits and lands into the disk.

Centerwatch—maintains a Web site that lists 7,000 (of the 70,000) current clinical trials in the U.S., many of which are recruiting participants

central processing unit (CPU)—contains the arithmetic-logic unit and control unit

Child Behavior Toolbox Professional—a database of strategies for therapists who work with children between the ages of two and 12 who have behavior and learning problems

chip—silicon chip on which thousands of microscopic circuits are burned

CINAHL—The Cumulative Index to Nursing and Allied Health Literature is an up-to-date database for nurses and allied health professionals

clearinghouse—a business that collects insurance claims from providers and sends them to the correct insurance carrier

clinical application—the use of information technology for direct patient care; includes patient monitoring, interventional radiology, surgery, and electronic prosthetics

clinical pharmacology—a database of the latest drug information

ClinicalTrials.gov—Web site that was launched in February 2000; it lists thousands of clinical trials along with their purpose, criteria for participation, location, and contact information

CMS-1500—HCFA-1500 (the most commonly accepted claim form) is being renamed CMS-1500.

code of conduct—internal company policy which attempts to safeguard information and guarantee privacy

communications software—applications software which allows the connection of one computer to other computers

Composite International Diagnostic Interview (CIDI)—a tool for diagnosing mental disorders

Composite International Diagnostic Interview-Auto—a computerized version of CIDI; can be self-administered

computer—an electronic device that can accept data (raw facts) as input, process or alter them in some way, and produce useful information as output

computer-assisted surgery—makes use of computers, robotic devices, and/or computer-generated images in the planning and carrying out of surgical procedures

computer-assisted trial design—software that allows the simulation of clinical drug trials before the actual trials begin

computer literacy—familiarity with and knowledge about computers, the Internet, and the World Wide Web; the ability to use computers to perform tasks in one's own field

computerized functional electrical stimulation (CFES or FES)—a technique involving the use of low-level electrical stimulation; has been used for many years in pacemakers and other implanted devices; now used to strengthen paralyzed muscles with simulated exercise; low-level electrical stimulation is applied directly to muscles that cannot receive these signals from the brain because of spinal cord injury

computerized medical instruments—contain microprocessors and provide direct patient services such as monitoring, administering medication, or treatment

computerized tomography (CT)—an imaging technique which involves taking a series of X-rays at different angles from which the computer constructs a cross-sectional image

connectivity—the fact that computers can be connected to each other

continuous speech recognition system—enables the computer to respond to commands or dictation spoken naturally; requires certain hardware and software.

control unit—the part of the central processing unit that controls processing following the instructions of a program; it directs the movement of electronic signals between parts of the computer

cookies—small files put on a user's hard drive when the user visits a Web site

cosmetic dentistry—branch of dentistry that attempts to create a more attractive smile; may use bonding, sculpting the gum line, tooth bleaching, and dental implants

corneal topography—uses a computer to create an accurate three-dimensional map of the cornea

Cumulative Index to Nursing and Allied Health Literature (CINAHL)—a database specifically geared to the needs of nurses and other professionals in 17 allied health fields, including dental hygiene, occupational therapy, and radiology; includes an index of 1,000 journals from 1982 to the present, bibliographic citations of books, pamphlets, software, and standards of practice, abstracts or full text of articles where they are available, journals and descriptions of Web sites of interest.

current procedures terminology (CPT)—codes lab tests, treatments, and other procedures

da Vinci—a surgical robot

data—raw facts

data accuracy—correctness and currency of information

Databank for Cardiovascular Disease—at Duke University, a highly specialized expert system that combines computer monitoring with extensive collections of information on cardiac patients

database—a large organized collection of information that is easy to maintain, search, and sort

database management system (DBMS)—application software which allows the user to enter organized lists of data and easily edit, sort, and search them

DBMS (database management system)—application software that allows the user to create, maintain, sort and search databases

demineralize—teeth are constantly affected by acids, that demineralize the surfaces; early lesions beneath the enamel can be treated with calcium, phosphate, and fluoride, which help remineralize teeth

diagnosis related group (DRG)—code used for diagnosis; hospital reimbursement by insurers is based on a formula using DRGs

DIFOTI®—Digital Imaging Fiber-Optic Trans-illumination (DIFOTI®) involves using a digital CCD camera to obtain images of teeth trans-illuminated with white light; images are analyzed using computer algorithms

digital device—a device that computes by counting; for example, a digital thermometer counts degrees of temperature

digital signal—a discontinuous pulse; an on or off; digital computers process digital signals

direct-entry devices—input devices including scanning and pointing devices, and sensors.

discrete speech recognition system—enables the computer to respond to commands or dictation; however, the user must pause between words

distance surgery (telepresence surgery)—surgery performed by robotic devices controlled by surgeons at another site

drill-and-practice software—educational programs that can repeat questions as many times as necessary; used in disciplines that require memorization, to teach such things as math facts or foreign languages

DVD (digital video disks)—high-capacity optical disks store data as pits and lands burnt by a laser into a plastic disk.

electrical conductance—electrical conductance is currently used to diagnose cavities; an electric current is passed through a tooth, and the tooth's resistance is measured

Electronic Communications Privacy Act of 1986—prohibits government agencies from intercepting electronic communications without a search warrant and prohibits individuals from intercepting e-mail; however, there are numerous exceptions and the courts have interpreted this to allow employers to access employees' e-mail; this law does not apply to communications within an organization

electronic mail (e-mail)—allows a user to send messages to another user's computer; fast, convenient, and inexpensive, but not private

electronic remittance advice (ERA)—accompanies the response to an electronically submitted claim

electronic spreadsheet—applications software that allows the user to store and manipulate numbers

EMC (electronic media claim)—is an electronically processed and transmitted claim

encounter form—superbill; list of diagnoses and procedures common to the practice; superbills for each patient on a day's schedule are printed that morning or the night before

encryption—used to protect information from unauthorized users, involves encoding of messages

endoscope—a thin tube with a light source that either allows a direct view into the body or is connected to a minuscule camera which projects an image of the surgical site onto a monitor

environmental control system—hardware and software that help physically challenged people control their environments

expansion boards—circuit boards that are plugged into the expansion slots on the main circuit board; they include the electronic circuitry needed by added-on hardware

expansion slots—slots in the main circuit board which allow expansion boards to be inserted.

expert system—a program that attempts to make computers mimic human expertise in limited fields; uses a database of numerous facts and rules about how decisions are made

EXPERTMD—software that allows the creation of medical and dental expert systems

explanation of benefits (EOB)—the insurance company's response to a paper claim that explains why certain services were covered and others not

explorable virtual human—is being developed. It will include authoring tools that engineers can use to build anatomical models that will allow students to experience how real anatomical structures feel, appear, and sound.

extranet—a corporate intranet connected to other intranets outside the corporation

facial structure scan—a biometric method that identifies users by facial structure

facial thermography—a biometric method that identifies users by the heat generated by their faces

Fair Credit Reporting Act of 1970—a federal law which regulates credit agencies; it allows you to see your credit reports to check the accuracy of information and to challenge inaccuracies

Fee-for-service plans—insurance plan in which patient is never restricted to a network of providers and needs no referrals for specialists; after fulfilling a deductible (a certain amount the patient is required to pay each year before the insurance begins paying,) every visit to a doctor is paid for by the insurance company

fetal monitor—measures fetal heart rate

fiber-optic transillumination—fiber-optic transillumination found early lesions (affecting enamel), but was limited in diagnosing advanced caries.

field—one piece of information about an item in a database table, for example, Social Security number or last name

file—a table in a database containing related records, for example, all doctors in a practice

fingerprint—biometric method of identification

firewall—software used to protect LANs from unauthorized access through the Internet

focused ultrasound surgery—in the early experimental stages; uses sound waves to raise the temperature of cancerous tissue until it dies; also being examined as a way to stop massive bleeding

Food and Drug Administration (FDA)—federal agency in charge of reviewing and approving new drugs

fraud—includes such crimes as using a computer program to illegally transfer money from one bank account to another, or printing payroll checks to oneself

functional electrical stimulation (FES or CFES)—see computerized functional electrical stimulation

gamma knife—bloodless surgical device, works by delivering 201 focused beams of radiation directly at a brain tumor, killing the tumor and sparing the surrounding tissue

gamma knife surgery—bloodless surgery using a gamma knife

GDx Access—uses an infrared laser to measure the thickness of the retinal nerve fiber. It is used for the early detection of glaucoma

graphical user interface (GUI)—an operating environment or interface used by Windows and Macintosh OS which allows users to interact with the computer by clicking on icons with a mouse

graphics software—applications software that allows the user to create graphics, from simple line graphs to presentations

guarantor—the person responsible for paying a medical bill after all insurance is received

hacker—unauthorized user

hand print—biometric method of identification used to restrict access to computers

hard copy—printed output

hardware—the physical components of a computer

HCFA-1500—the most widely accepted claim form (currently being renamed CMS-1500)

HCPCS (Healthcare Common Procedure Coding Systems)—developed to standardize claims processing for government and private insurance; divided into three subsystems

head mouse—input device that moves the cursor according to the user's head motions

Health Care Financing Administration (HCFA)—several government insurance plans administered by the federal Health Care Financing Administration (HCFA); renamed Centers for Medicaid and Medicare Services (CMS)

Health Insurance Portability and Accountability Act of 1996—first federal privacy protection of personally identifiable medical information; encourages the use of the electronic medical record.

health maintenance organization (HMO)—insurance in which patient pays a fixed yearly fee and must choose among an approved network of health care providers and hospitals

Healthcare Common Procedure Coding Systems (HCPCS)—developed to standardize claims processing for government and private insurance; divided into three systems

Healthfinder—(http://www.healthfinder.gov), a listing of "sites 'hand-picked' . . . by health professionals"

Heidelberg Retinal Tomograph (HRT)—uses lasers to scan the retina, resulting in a three-dimensional description

HERMES—an FDA-cleared computer operating system that controls all the electronic equipment in the operating room, coordinating the endoscope and robotic devices

HMO (health maintenance organization)—insurance in which a patient pays a fixed yearly fee, and must choose among an approved network of health care providers and hospitals

Homeland Security Act (2002)—expands and centralizes the data gathering allowed under the U.S.A. Patriot Act

Human Genome Project—international project (begun in 1990) seeking to understand the human genetic makeup; to find the 100,000 or so human genes and to read the entire genetic script, all 3 billion bits of information, by the year 2005

human-biology input device—uses sensors to interpret body movements and characteristics, allowing the user's body to be used as an input device

ICD-9-CM (International Classification of Disease)—classifies diseases using 4-5 digit codes

identity theft—involves someone using your private information to assume your identity

ILIAD—a program that provides hypothetical cases for the student to evaluate; the student's diagnostic abilities are then compared to the computer's

image-guided surgery—surgery guided by computer-generated images of the surgical field, not a direct view

impact printer—a printer that creates hard copy by having a print head strike a ribbon and the paper; includes dot-matrix printer

indemnity plan—insurance in which the patient is never restricted to a network of providers and needs no referrals for specialists; after fulfilling a deductible (a certain amount the patient is required to pay each year before the insurance begins paying), every visit to a doctor is paid for by the insurance company

information technology (IT)—includes computers, communications networks, and computer literacy

input device—a device that translates data into a form the computer can process (bits)

insertion point—indicates where the next character typed will go

interactive videoconferencing (teleconferencing)—allows doctors and patients to consult in real time, at a distance

International Classification of Disease (ICD-9-CM)—codes thousands of diseases using 4-5 digit codes

Internet (interconnected network)—a global network of networks, connecting innumerable smaller networks, computers, and users

Internet service provider (ISP)—a company that sells a user a temporary connection to the Internet

INTERNIST—medical expert system used as decision support system to help in diagnosis

interventional radiology—the use of the tools of radiology to treat conditions that once required surgery

intranet—a private corporate network that uses the same structure as the Internet and TCP/IP protocols

intra-oral fiber-optic camera—allows both patient and dentist to get a close-up tour of the patient's mouth.

iris scan—a biometric method of identification used to restrict access to computers

keyboard—an input device

KISMET—simulation software used in surgery

Kurzweil scanner—a direct-entry input device, scanning device; scans printed text and reads it aloud to the user

laparoscope—endoscope used for abdominal surgery

laser—light amplification by stimulated emission of radiation; lasers deliver light energy; depending on the target, the light travels at different wavelengths.

LASIK—eye surgery performed with lasers, which corrects vision and makes glasses less necessary

line-of-sight system—allows you to use your body as an input device; the user's eyes can point to a part of the screen; a camera and computer can identify the area you are looking at

lip print—biometric method of identification used to restrict access to computers

local area networks (LAN)—small private networks that span one room or building

magnetic disk—storage medium that stores data as magnetic spots

magnetic resonance imaging (MRI)—an imaging technique that uses computer technology to produce images of soft tissue within the body that could not be pictured by traditional X-rays; can produce images of the insides of bones; uses computers and a very strong magnetic field and radio waves to generate mathematical data from which an image is constructed

magnetic tape—secondary storage medium; sequential access storage

managed care—insurance in which it is the insurance carrier that determines what treatment is necessary and pays for it; there are several forms of managed care where patients pay a fixed yearly fee, and the insurance company pays the participating provider

Medicaid—jointly funded, federal-state health insurance for certain low-income and needy people

medical informatics—the use of technology to organize information in health care

Medical Information Bureau—comprised of 650 insurance companies, its database contains health histories of millions of people; used by medical insurers to help determine insurance rates and whether to grant or deny someone medical coverage; not protected by doctor-patient privilege, and at present do not know the effect HIPAA will have

Medicare—federal insurance that serves people 65 and over and disabled people with chronic renal disorders; allows patients to choose their physicians; referrals are not needed

MediSoft—software used for managing a medical office

MediSoft Patient Aging Report—report used to show a patient's outstanding payments; current and past due balances are listed on this report based on the number of days late

MEDI-SPAN—a database of information on drug/drug and drug/food interactions

MEDLARS (Medical Literature Analysis and Retrieval System)—a collection of 40 computerized databases containing 18 million references, available free via the Internet; can be searched for bibliographical lists or for information

MEDLINE—a comprehensive online database of current medical research, including publications from 1966 to the present; contains 8.5 million articles from 3700 journals; 31,000 citations are added each month

MEDLINEPlus—an online medical database for consumers

memory—temporary storage area used during processing; internal storage made up of RAM and ROM

mental health aide—a self-administered psychiatric interview that prints out reports on symptoms, current stress, psychiatric history, and other relevant data

MINERVA—a robot developed to perform stereotactic neurosurgical procedures

minimally invasive dentistry—emphasizes prevention and the least possible intervention

minimally invasive surgery (MIS)—surgery performed through small incisions

minimum data set—resident assessment instruments used to assess each patient in a nursing home and to assign each to one of seven categories of resource utilization groups

monitor—screen

motherboard—main circuit board of the computer; also called system board

mouse—a direct-entry input device; pointing device, used to select items from a menu and position the insertion point

MYCIN—an expert system used as a decision support system to help in the diagnosis and treatment of bacterial infections

myoelectric limbs—artificial limbs containing motors and responding to the electrical signals transmitted by the residual limb to electrodes mounted in the socket

neonatal monitor—monitors infant heart and breathing rates

network—computers and other hardware devices linked together via communications media

New Medicines in Development—a database that provides information on newly approved drugs and drugs awaiting approval

open architecture—computer design that allows hardware devices to be added by plugging expansion boards into expansion slots on the main circuit board

operating system—the system software that controls the basic operation of the computer hardware, managing the resources of the computer including input and output, the execution of programs, and processor time; provides the user interface

optical disk—secondary storage device on which data is represented by pits and lands burnt in by a laser

optical biometry—in cataract surgery, the eye's lens is replaced by an intra-ocular lens. The measurements used to determine which IOL to use are determined by calculations referred to as optical biometry

Optomap Panoramic 200—can examine the retina without dilation using low-powered red and green lasers

output devices—hardware that presents information in a form a human user can comprehend

pages—the Web is made up of documents called pages

page scanner—a direct-entry input device that digitizes printed text

Palmtops (personal digital assistants)—handheld computers

password—a secret code assigned to (or chosen by) an authorized user

patient aging report—used to show a patient's outstanding payments; current and past due balances are listed on this report based on the number of days late

patient day sheet—report that lists the day's patients

payment day sheet—a grouped report organized by providers; each patient is listed under his or her provider; report shows the amounts received from each patient to each provider

Payments—amounts received by providers

PediaSim—a programmable mannequin of a child; used for teaching

personal identification number (PIN)—a secret code assigned to (or chosen by) an authorized user

physiological monitoring systems—systems that monitor physiological processes; analyze blood and other fluids

Physiome Project—project attempting to develop accurate and complete human physiological models, which may in the future be used as simulated patients in drug trials

PLATO—an early simulation program; as early as 1963, computer-based nursing courses were developed using PLATO (Programmed Logic for Automatic Teaching Operations)

plotter—output device that produces hard copy; used for graphics, such as maps and architectural drawings

port—a socket on the outside of the computer

positron emission tomography (PET)—an imaging technique that uses radioisotope technology to create a picture of the body "in action"; uses computers to construct images from the emission of positive electrons (positrons) by radioactive substances administered to the patient

Post Operative Expert Medical System (POEMS)—an expert system that focuses on patients who become sick while recovering from surgery

practice—a group of health care practitioners in business together

practice analysis report—generated on a monthly basis; a summary total of all procedures, charges, and transactions

preferred provider organization (PPO)—insurance that allows patient to seek care within an approved network of health care providers who have agreed with the insurance company to lower their charges and accept assignment (the amount the insurance company pays)

printer—output device that produces hard copy

privacy—the ability to control personal information and the right to keep it from misuse

procedure day sheet—a grouped report organized by procedure; patients who underwent a particular procedure such as a blood sugar lab test are listed under that procedure

processor (system unit)—contains the CPU and memory; does the actual manipulation of data

program—step-by-step instructions; also called software

Programmed Logic for Automatic Teaching Operations (PLATO)—an early CAI program used in the education of nurses

prosthetic devices—replacement limbs and organs

protocols—technical standards governing communication between computers

puff straw—an input device that allows people to control the mouse with their mouths

pulmonary monitor—monitoring system that measures blood flow through the heart and respiratory rate

random access memory (RAM)—the part of temporary, volatile internal storage that holds the work you are currently doing while you are doing it, including the program and data you are using; the operating system must be in RAM for other programs to run

rational drug design—a technique that utilizes computers to model molecules and develop chemical compunds which will bind to the target molecule and inhibit or stimulate it; used in the development of drugs that are used for Alzheimer's, hypertension, and AIDS

read only memory (ROM)—part of internal memory; firmware; permanent instructions that the user normally cannot change

record—a collection of related fields; all the information on one item in a database table

relational database—an organized collection of related data; information input in one part of the program can be linked to information in another part of the program; a collection of tables related by common fields

remineralize—early lesions beneath the enamel can be treated with calcium, phosphate, and fluoride, which help remineralize teeth (restore the enamel)

remote monitoring device—a monitoring device that transmits signals over communications lines, making it possible for patients to be monitored at home or in ambulances

resource utilization groups (RUGs)—system that bases payment on average prices, with adjustments

retina scan—a biometric method of identifying users

ribonucleic acid (RNA)—made in the nucleus of a cell, but not restricted to the nucleus; long coiled-up molecule whose purpose is to take the blueprint from DNA and build our actual proteins

RNA interference (RNAi)—a process that cells use to turn off genes; the attempt at developing drugs based on RNAi is in its infancy,

ROBODOC—a computer-controlled, image-directed robot used in hip-replacement surgery

robot—a programmable machine that can manipulate its environment

scanning devices—translate printed material into bits

schedule of benefits—a list of those services that the insurance carrier will cover

scientific visualization—the process of graphically representing the results of numerical calculations

screen reader software—software that tells the speech synthesizer what to say, for example, to read the text description of an icon

SDILINE (Selective Dissemination of Information onLINE)—contains only the latest month's additions to MEDLINE

search engine—software that allows you to search the Web

secondary storage devices—include disk drives and tape drives, which, with their media, allow the more permanent storage of data, programs, and information than primary storage

security—measures attempting to protect computer systems (including hardware, software, and information), from harm and abuse; the threats may stem from many sources including natural disaster, human error, or crime

sensor—a direct-entry input device that collects data directly from the environment and sends it to a computer; used to collect patient information for clinical monitoring systems

simulation software—educational software that attempts to recreate a real situation

SOCRATES—a long-distance mentoring system; cleared by the FDA in 2001

soft copy—output on a monitor or voice output

software (programs)—the step-by-step instructions that tell the computer what to do

software piracy—unauthorized copying of copyrighted software

speaker-dependent—speech recognition system that needs to be trained to recognize the user's speech patterns

speaker-independent—speech recognition system that recognizes a limited number of commands spoken in standard North American English

special purpose application—the use of information technology for applications not included in clinical or adminstrative applications. These include drug design and education

SPECT (single photon emission computed tomography)—an imaging technique that, like the PET scan, shows movement; less precise and less expensive than PET

speech recognition—enables the computer to respond to spoken commands or dictation

speech synthesizer—a device with a processor, memory, and output capability, which turns digital data into speechlike sounds, allowing the computer to talk

Starbright World—a network linking seriously ill children in 100 hospitals in the United States (1998); children in the networked hospitals can play games, chat, send and receive e-mail, and receive medical information

stereotactic radiosurgery—gamma knife surgery; used to treat brain tumors

store-and-forward technology—technique in which the data to be sent is digitized, stored, and transmitted over a telecommunications network

superbill (encounter form)—list of diagnoses and procedures common to the practice; superbills for each patient on a day's schedule are printed that morning or the night before.

system board—motherboard; main circuit board of the computer

system software—programs that control hardware operations and interact between the applications and the computer; includes the operating system, utility programs, and language translators

system unit—processor that contains the CPU and memory

table—a collection of related records in a database file

TCP/IP (transmission control protocol/Internet Protocol)—standards governing the Internet

telecommuting—involves working at home on computers linked by telecommunications lines to one's office

teleconferencing—may involve anything from a conference call to a meeting between people who are not in the same place, but who can see and hear each other via video and audio equipment; it may also involve sharing documents on monitors and being able to work on them cooperatively.

teledentistry—teledentistry programs have been developed to help dentists access specialists, improving patient care

telehealth—includes telemedicine and other health-related activities using telecommunications lines and computers, including education, research, public health, and administration of health services

telehome care—involves the monitoring of vital signs from a distance via telecommunications equipment, and the replacement of home nursing visits with videoconferences; usually used to manage chronic conditions such as congestive heart failure and diabetes

telemedicine—the delivery of health care over telecommunications lines

telenurse—a nurse who practices over telecommunications lines

teleoncology—the use of telemedicine in the treatment of cancer

telepathology—the transmission of microscopic images over telecommunications lines

telepharmacy—the linking of the prescribing doctor's office with the dispensing pharmacy via telecommunications lines

telepresence surgery (distance surgery)—surgery performed by robotic devices controlled by surgeons at another site

telepsychiatry—the delivery of therapy using teleconferencing

teleradiology—the sending of radiological images in digital form over telecommunications lines

telespirometry—monitoring system used by asthmatic patients; designed to transmit over the telephone to a remote location

teletriage—telemedicine application in which calls are screened

text telephone—allows people to communicate on the phone using keyboards and printers

theft of information—unauthorized access to and use of information

theft of services—unauthorized use of services such as cable TV

tonometers—measure eye pressure

Total Information Awareness Program—a program that would allow government to link private and public databases; so far has not passed into law

transactions—charges, payments, and adjustments

transmission control protocol/Internet protocol (TCP/IP)—the protocol that governs the Internet

TRICARE—federal health benefits program that supplements medical care in the military

ultrafast CT—a variation of the traditional CT scan; may be used in place of a coronary angiogram to examine coronary artery blockages; compared with a coronary angiogram, the ultrafast CT is painless, less dangerous, noninvasive, and less expensive.

ultrasound—an imaging technique that uses no radiation; uses very high frequency sound waves and the echoes they produce when they hit an object to generate information that is used by a computer to create a two-dimensional moving image on a screen; used to examine a moving fetus, to study blood flow, and to diagnose gallstones and prostate disease.

uniform resource locator (URL)—address of a Web page

USA Patriot Act (2001)—gives law enforcement agencies greater power to monitor electronic and other communications, with fewer checks

user interface (operating environment)—defines how the user communicates with the computer

virtual environment—technology used to provide surgeons with realistic accurate models on which to teach surgery and plan and practice operations

Virtual Hospital—a comprehensive and authoritative Web site that has been maintained by the University of Iowa since 1992; its information (available for patients and health care providers) comes from 350 peer-reviewed sources

Virtual Human Embryo—A new project that is digitizing some of the 7,000 human embryos lost in miscarriages, which have been kept by the National Museum of Health and Medicine of the Armed Forces Institute of Pathology since the 1880s; an embryo develops in 23 stages over the first eight weeks of pregnancy, and the project will include at least one embryo from each stage

virtual reality (VR)—technology that allows the computer to create an environment that seems real, but is not; used in planning and teaching surgical and other procedures

virus—a program, attached to another file, which replicates itself and may do damage to your computer system

visual function analyzer—measures how well you can see by measuring how your eye focuses light

Visible Human Project—a computerized library of human anatomy at the National Library of Medicine, seeking to create accurate, three-dimensional representations of the male and female body; the project began in the late 1980s and now contains images of 1,800 cross-sections of a male cadaver (39 years old) and 5,000 of a female cadaver (59 years old) accessible over the Internet

Web browser—software needed to browse the Web

Web sites—files in which information on the Web are stored

wide area network (WAN)—a network that may span a state, country, or even the world

word processing software—application software that allows the user to create, edit, format, save, retrieve, and print text documents

workers' compensation—a government program that covers job-related illness or injury

World Wide Web (Web or WWW)—the part of the Internet that is most accessible and easiest to navigate, organized as sites with hyperlinks to one another

X-ray—a traditional imaging technique that uses high-energy electromagnetic waves to produce a two-dimensional picture on film; does not produce good images of all organs and cannot see behind bones

ZEUS—"a robotic surgical system which makes possible minimally invasive microsurgery; has three interactive robotic arms, one of which holds the endoscope, while the other two manipulate the surgical instruments; the surgeon, sitting at a console, controls them; includes a feedback system so that the surgeon feels the tissue"

Index

A

Accounting, 46, 51
  using MediSoft, 46
Accounting reports, 51
  patient aging report, 51
  patient day sheet, 51
  payment day sheet, 51
  prodecure day sheet, 51
Accounts receivable (A/R), 50
ADA. *see* American Dental Association
ADAM, 177, 178; *see also* Simulation software
Adaptive technology, 156, 158–62; *see also*
    Assistive technology
ADE. *see* Adverse drug event
Adjustments, 46
Administrative applications, 42, 43–44
  in dentistry, 97–100
  electronic dental chart, 97–100
  electronic medical record, 208–10
  office management, 43–44
Administrative software, 44–46
  coding, 46
  electronic medical record (EMR),
    45–46, 208–10
  grouping, 46
  patient information form, 45
Advanced Research Projects Agency of the
    U.S. Department of Defense
    (ARPA), 9, 123
Adverse drug event (ADE), 139
AESOP, 119, 120, 123; *see also* Surgery
AI. *see* Artificial intelligence
AIDSLINE, 10, 187; *see also* Medical
    literature databases
Ambulatory patient classification (APC),
    51–52

American Dental Association (ADA), 97
American Medical Association (AMA), 194,
    208
Americans with Disabilities Act of 1990, 158
Analog device, 3–4; *see also* Hardware
Analog signal, 9
Antisense technology, 137
APC. *see* Ambulatory patient classification
Applications
  administrative, 42, 43–44, 208–10
  clinical, 42
  special purpose, 42
Application software, 7–8; *see also* Software
Arithmetic-logic unit, 5–6
ARPAnet, 9–10
Arrhythmia monitoring, 65, 157; *see also*
    Remote monitoring devices
ARTEMIS, 122; *see also* Surgery
Artificial intelligence, 116
Assignment, 47
Assistive devices, 158–64
  augmentative communications devices,
    160–61; *see also* Assistive devices
  environmental control systems, 161–62
  head mouse, 160
  prosthetic devices, 162–64
  puff straws, 160
  speech recognition, 159–60
  text telephones, 160
Assistive technology, 156, 158–62; *see also*
    Adaptive technology
Augmentative communication device,
    160–62; *see also* Assistive devices
Augmented reality surgery, 116, 122; *see*
    also Computer-assisted surgery
Authorization, 47
Automatic recalculation, 7

B

Baby CareLink, 67
Balance billing, 43, 50; *see also* Bucket billing
Balanced Budget Act of 1997, 51, 69
Bar codes, hospital pharmacy, 142, 143
Binary digit (bit), 3
Bioinformatics, 135
Biometric keyboards, 24; *see also* Biometric
     methods of restricting access
Biometrics, 5
Biometric methods of restricting access,
     24–25; *see also* Security
  biometric keyboards, 24
  body odor sensors, 24
  facial structure scans, 25
  facial thermography, 24
  fingerprints, 24
  hand prints, 24
  iris scans, 24
  lip prints, 24
  retina scans, 24
Biomicroscopes, 158
Biotechnology, 134–37
  developments in, 136–37
Bit, 3
Bloodless surgery, 80, 86–87
  gamma knife surgery, 80, 86–87
  focused ultrasound, 87
  stereotactic radiosurgery, 86
Bluetooth, 8, 63
Body odor sensors, 24; *see also* Biometric
     methods of restricting access
Bonding, 103, 103; *see also* Cosmetic
     dentistry
Bone density (DEXA) scans, 86; *see also*
     Digital imaging techniques
Boot, 7
Bucket billing, 43, 50; *see also* Balance billing

C

Cable modem, 9
Capitated plan, 48
Case, 46
CD (compact disk), 6; *see also* Secondary
     storage media
Centers for Medicare and Medicaid
     Services (CMS), 45, 47, 48

Centerwatch, 187; *see also* Medical literature
     databases
Central processing unit (CPU), 5; *see also*
     Processing hardware
CFES. *see* Computerized functional electri-
     cal stimulation
CHAMPVA, 47
Charges, 46
Children's Online Privacy Protection Act
     of 2000, 23
Chip, 3
CINAHL (The Cumulative Index to Nursing
     and Allied Health Literature), 189;
     see also Medical literature databases
Claims, 48–50; *see also* Insurance
Clearinghouse, 48
C-leg, 162–63
Clinical applications, 42
  future trends in, 206–208
Clinical pharmacology, 187; *see also*
     Medical literature databases
ClinicalTrials.gov, 187; *see also* Medical
     literature databases
CMS-1500, 48; *see also* HCFA-1500
Codes of conduct, 22; *see also* Security
Coding, 46; *see also* Administrative
     software; Grouping systems
Communications, 8–9, 160–62; *see also*
     Telecommunications
  hardware, 9; *see also* Hardware
    modem, 9
  software, 8; *see also* Software
Compact disk (CD), 6; *see also* Secondary
     storage media
Computer(s)
  and crime, 21–22
  defined, 2
  drug errors and, 138–39
  federal legislation on, 23–24
  literacy, information technology (IT)
     and, 2
  in the medical office, 43ff.
Computer Abuse Amendments Act (1994),
     23
Computer-aided design and manufacturing
     (CAD/CAM), 103, 162
Computer-assisted
  drug review, 138
  drug trials, 137

instruction (CAI), 177ff.; *see also*
  Education
surgery, 116–26; *see also* Surgery
  augmented reality, 122
  and robotics, 118
  surgical planning, 116–17
  trial design (CATD), 137
Computer Fraud and Abuse Act of 1984, 23
Computer literacy, 2
Computer Matching and Privacy
  Protection Act of 1988, 23
Computerized functional electrical stimu-
  lation (CFES), 156, 165–66
Computerized instruments in dentistry,
  102
Computerized medical instruments, 156–58
  in optometry/ophthalmology, 157–58
Computerized pharmacies, 138–43
Computerized tomography (CT), 80, 82–83;
  see also Digital imaging techniques
Confidential Information Protection Act
  of 2001, 24
Connectivity, overview of, 8–9
Consumer Internet Privacy Enhancement
  Act of 2001, 24
Continuous speech recognition systems, 159
Control unit, 6
Cookies, 26
Copayment, 47
Corneal topography, 158
Cosmetic dentistry, 103
CPT (*Current Procedural Terminology*), 46; *see
  also* Coding
Crime, computer technology and, 21–22
Current Procedural Terminology. see CPT

D

Data, 2
Data accuracy, 21
Databank for Cardiovascular Disease, 186;
  see also Expert systems
Database management system (DBMS), 7, 44
Databases, 26–29, 44
  file, 44
  government, 27–28
  and the Internet, 29
  medical literature, 187–89
  in the medical office, 43–44

private, 28–29
privacy and, 29–32, 32–33
Da Vinci system, 121; *see also* Minimally
  invasive surgery (MIS)
Deductible, 47
Demineralize, 108
Demographic changes and occupational
  outlook, 210–11
Demographic changes and dentistry,
  100–102
Dental implants, 103; *see also* Cosmetic
  dentistry
Dental informatics, 96
Dentistry, 95–111
  administrative applications, 97–100
  computerized instruments in, 102
  cosmetic, 103
  demographics and, 100–102
  diagnosis in, 103–106
  diagnostic tools, 104–106
  education, 96–97
  endodontics, 102–103
  expert systems, 103–104
  growth of specialization in, 109
  lasers in, 106–108
  minimally invasive, 108
  periodontics, 103
  surgery in, 109
  transformation of, 100–102
DentSim, 97
DEXA (bone density) scan, 86
Diagnosis related group. *see* DRG
Diagnosis in dentistry, 103–106
Diagnostic tools, used in dentistry, 104–106
Digital device, 3–4; *see also* Hardware
Digital Imaging Fiber-Optic
  Transillumination (DIFOTI®), 106,
  107, 110
Digital imaging techniques, 82–86
  bone density (DEXA) scans, 86
  computerized tomography (CT), 82–83
  fMRI, 83–84
  magnetic resonance imaging (MRI), 80,
  83–84
  positron emission tomography (PET),
  84–85
  SPECT (single photon emission computed tomography), 82
Digital radiography, 81, 104

Digital video disk (DVD), 6; *see also* Secondary storage media
Digital signals, 9
Digitize, 3
Direct-entry devices, 4; *see also* Input device
Discrete speech recognition systems, 159
Distance learning, 181, 185; *see also* Education
Distance (telepresence) surgery, 116, 123
Doctor's Book of Home Remedies, 195
DRG (diagnosis related group), 46; *see also* Grouping
Driver Privacy Protection Act, 23
Driver's License Modernization Act, 4
Drug delivery on a chip, 145
Drug dispensing, point-of-use, 142–43
Drug distribution systems, automated, 140–43
  in community pharmacies, 140–41
  in hospital pharmacies, 142–43
Drug errors, computers and, 138–39
Drug review, computer-assisted, 138
Drug trials, computer-assisted, 137
DVD (digital video disk), 6; *see also* Secondary storage media

E

Education, 176–85
  computer-assisted instruction (CAI), 177
  in dentistry, 96–97
  distance learning, 181, 185
  patient simulators, 181, 182–84
    Pedia-Sim, 181
  simulation software, 178
  virtual reality simulations, 178–81
  Visible Human Project, 176–77
Electrical conductance, 106
Electronic Communications Privacy Act of 1986, 23, 25
Electronic dental chart, 97–100
Electronic medical record (EMR), 45–46, 208–10; *see also* Administrative applications
  privacy and, 32–33
Electronic Privacy Protection Act of 2001, 24
Electronic remittance advice (ERA), 48; *see also* Claims

Electronic spreadsheets, 7
E-mail, 8, 32, 189–92
  health information via, 189–92
  privacy and, 32
EMC (electronic media claim), 48; *see also* Claims
Emerging methods in dentistry, 106
EMR. *see* Electronic medical record
Encounter form, 46, 50; *see also* Superbill
Encryption, 22; *see also* Security
Endodontics, 102–103
Endoscope, 102, 116, 117, 119, 120–21
Environmental control systems, 161–62; *see also* Assistive devices
Expansion boards, 6
Expansion slots, 6
EXPERTMD, 104
Expert systems, 185–86, 103–104
  Databank for Cardiovascular Disease, 186
  dentistry, 103–104
  INTERNIST, 185–86
  MYCIN, 185
  Post Operative Expert Medical System (POEMS), 186
Explanation of benefits (EOB), 48; *see also* Claims
Explorable virtual human, 177
Extranet, 10

F

Facial structure scans, 25; *see also* Biometic methods of restricting access
Facial thermography, 24; *see also* Biometric methods of restricting access
Fair Credit Reporting Act of 1970, 23, 29
  Amendments of 2001, 24
FDA. *see* Food and Drug Administration
Federal legislation on computers and privacy, 23–24
Fee-for-service plans, 47
Fetal monitors, 157
Fiber-optic camera, 102, 106
Fiber-optic transillumination, 106
Fields, 44
Fingerprints, 24; *see also* Biometric methods of restricting access

Firewall, 10, 25; *see also* Security
Focused ultrasound surgery, 87; *see also* Bloodless surgery
Food and Drug Administration (FDA), 65, 69, 81, 118, 119, 122, 136–37, 138, 146–47, 164
Fraud, 21
Functional MRIs, 83–84, 85; *see also* Digital imaging techniques
Future trends, 206–208

G

Gamma knife surgery, 80, 86–7; *see also* Bloodless surgery
GDx Access, 158
Given® Diagnostic Imaging System, 85
Government databases, 27–28; *see also* Databases
Graphical user interface, 7
Graphics software, 7
Grouping systems, 46; *see also* Administrative software and coding systems
Guarantor, 47

H

Hackers, 33
Hand prints, 24; *see also* Biometric methods of restricting access
Hard copy, 6
Hardware, 3–6, 9
  analog devices, 3–4
  communications, 9
  digital devices, 3–4
  input devices, 4–5
  memory, 5–6
  open architecture, 6
  output devices, 6
  processing, 5–6
  secondary storage devices, 6
  secondary storage media, 6
HCFA-1500, 48, 49; *see also* CMS-1500
Head mouse, 160; *see also* Assistive devices
Health care
  privacy and, 29–33
  security and, 29–33
Healthcare Common Procedure Coding Systems (HCPCS), 52

Health Care Financing Administration (HCFA), 45, 48
Healthfinder, 11
Health information on the Internet, 186–95
  and e-mail, 189–92
  medical literature databases, 187–89
  reliability of, 194–95
Health Insurance Portability and Accountability Act (HIPAA) of 1996, 21, 23, 29, 30–31, 31–32, 33, 69
  privacy of medical records under, 31–32
Health maintenance organization (HMO), 48
Heidelberg Retinal Tomograph (HRT), 158
HERMES, 122; *see also* Computer-assisted surgery
HGP. *see* Human Genome Project
HHRG (Home Health Resource Group), 52
HIPAA. *see* Health Insurance Portability and Accountability Act of 1996
HMO. *see* Health maintenance organization (HMO)
Homeland Security Act of 2002, 23, 27–28
Hospital pharmacy, 142
  automating, 142
  bar codes, 142
  point-of-use drug dispensing, 142–43
  robot, 142
HPS. *see* Human patient simulators
Human Genome Project (HPG), 134–37
Human patient simulators (HPS), 181–84
Human-biology input device, 5; *see also* Input device

I

ICD-9-CM (*International Classification of Diseases Clinical Modification,* 9th edition), 46; *see also* Coding
Identity theft, 22
ILIAD, 178; *see also* Simulation software
Implants, risks posed by, 166
Indemnity plan, 47
Information, 2
Information technology (IT), 1–11
  computer literacy, 2

Information technology (*cont.*)
   in dentistry, 95–111
   in pharmacy, 133–48
      impact of, 145–46
   in radiology, 79–89
   in surgery, 115–27
   threats to, 21–25
Input devices, 4–5; *see also* Hardware
   direct-entry, 4
      scanning, 4
         bar-code, 4
         optical mark recognition (OMR), 4
         optical character recognition
           (OCR), 4
         magnetic ink character recognition
           (MICR), 4
      sensors, 5
      human-biology, 5
      keyboards, 4
      speech input, 5
Insertion point, 4
Insurance, 47–50
   claims, 48–50
Interactive videoconferencing (teleconfer-
   encing), 61, 62, 64, 65, 66, 68
Internal Revenue Service (IRS), 27
Internet, 2, 9–11; *see also* World Wide Web
   (WWW)
   databases and the, 29
   health information on, 186–95
   self-help on the, 192–93
   services, 10
   support groups, 193
Internet service provider (ISP), 10
INTERNIST, 185; *see also* Expert
   systems
Interventional radiology, 86; *see also*
   Bloodless surgery
Intranet, 10
Intra-oral fiber-optic cameras, 106
Iris scans, 24; *see also* Biometric methods of
   restricting access
IT. *see* Information technology (IT)

J

Journal of the American Medical Association
   (*JAMA*), 186, 189

K

Keyboards, 4; *see also* Input device
Key field, 44
KISMET, 122, 178; *see also* Surgery; Virtual
   reality simulations

L

Lasers, 106–108, 124
   in dentistry, 106–108
   in optometry/ophthalmology, 157–58
   in surgery, 124
LASIK surgery, 124; *see also* Surgery
Learning, distance, 181, 185
Learning Center for Interactive
   Technology, 181
Light illumination, 106
Lip prints, 24; *see also* Biometric methods
   of restricting access
Local area networks (LANs), 8

M

Magnetic disk, 6; *see also* Secondary storage
   media
Magnetic resonance imaging (MRI), 80,
   83–84; *see also* Digital imaging
   techniques
   functional (fMRI), 83–84; *see also* Digital
      imaging techniques
Magnetic tape, 6; *see also* Secondary storage
   media
Managed care, 47–48
Mayo Clinic Family Health Book on CR-ROM,
   195
Medicaid, 47
Medical HouseCall, 195
Medical informatics, 42
Medical Information Bureau, 28–29
Medical instruments, computerized,
   156–58
Medical literature databases, 187–89
   AIDSLINE, 10, 187
   Centerwatch, 187–88
   clinical pharmacology, 187
   ClinicalTrials.gov, 187
   CINAHL, 189
   MediSpan, 187

MEDLARS (Medical Literature Analysis and Retrieval System), 187
MEDLINE, 10, 187, 190, 194
New Medicines in Development, 187
PubMed, 10, 187, 190
SDILINE (Selective Dissemination of Information Online), 187
Medical office administrative software, 44–46
Medicare, 47
MediSoft, 7, 43, 50
  accounting using, 46
MediSpan, 187; *see also* Medical literature databases
MEDLARS (Medical Literature Analysis and Retrieval System), 187; *see also* Medical literature databases
MEDLINE, 10, 187, 190, 194; *see also* Medical literature databases
Memory, 5–6; *see also* Hardware
  random access memory (RAM), 6
  read only memory (ROM), 6
MINERVA, 121–22; *see also* Computer-assisted surgery
Minimally invasive dentistry, 108
Minimally invasive surgery (MIS), 116, 117–18; *see also* Computer-assisted surgery
Minimum data sets, 51
Modem, 9; *see also* Communications hardware
Monitoring devices, 65, 156–157
  computerized, 156–57
  remote, 65; *see also* Telemedicine
Monitors, 6; *see also* Output devices
Motherboard, 5; *see also* System board
Mouse, 4; *see also* Input device
MYCIN, 185; *see also* Expert systems
Myoelectric limbs, 162

N

National Information Infrastructure Protection Act of 1996, 23
Neonatal monitors, 157
Net. *see* Internet
Networking, 8–11
  overview of, 8–9
  protocols, 9
  uses of, 9

Networks, 2, 8
New Medicines in Development, 187; *see also* Medical literature databases

O

OASIS (Outcome and Assessment Information Set), 52
Occupational outlook for health care professionals, 210–11
Online Privacy Protection Act of 2001, 24
Open architecture, 6; *see also* Hardware
Operating system, 7
Optical biometry, 158
Optical disks, 6; *see also* Secondary storage media
Optical mark recognition (OMR), 4; *see also* Input devices
Optomap Panoramic200, 157–58
Optometry/ophthalmology, computerized devices in, 157–58
Output devices, 3, 6; *see also* Hardware
  monitors, 6
  plotters, 6
  printers, 6

P

Page scanners, 159
Passwords, 24; *see also* Security
Patient aging report, 51; *see also* Accounting reports
Patient day sheet, 51; *see also* Accounting reports
Patient information form, 45; *see also* Administrative software
Patient simulators, 178, 181, 182, 183, 184; *see also* Education
  PediaSim, 181, 182
Payment day sheet, 51; *see also* Accounting reports
Payments, 46
PediaSim, 181, 182; *see also* Patient simulators
Periodontics, 103
Personal Information Privacy Act of 2001, 24
Pharmacy, 133–48
  community, automated, 140–41

Pharmacy (*cont.*)
   computerized, 138–43
   computers and drug errors in, 138–39
   drug delivery on a chip, 145
   hospital, automated, 142–43
   impact of information technology on, 145–46
   point-of-use drug dispensing, 142–43
   telepharmacy, 143–45
   use of robots in, 140–41, 142
Pharmacology, clinical, 187; *see also* Medical literature databases
Physiological monitoring systems, 157
Physiome Project, 137
PINs (personal identification numbers), 24; *see also* Security
PLATO (Programmed Logic for Automatic Teaching Operations), 178
Plotters, 6; *see also* Output devices
Point-of-use drug dispensing, 142–43
Port, 6
Positron emission tomography (PET), 80, 82, 84–85; *see also* Digital imaging techniques
Post Operative Expert Medical System (POEMS), 186; *see also* Expert systems
Practice, 44
Practice analysis report, 51; *see also* Accounting reports
Preferred provider organizations (PPOs), 47
Printers, 6; *see also* Output devices
Privacy, 29–30, 30–33
   databases and, 26–29
   electronic medical records and, 32–33
   e-mail and, 32
   federal legislation on, 23–24, 30–32
   health care and, 29–33
   of medical records under HIPAA and the USA Patriot Act, 31–32
   overview of, 20–21
   telemedicine and, 32
Privacy Act (1974), 23
Private databases, 28–29; *see also* Databases
Procedure day sheet, 51; *see also* Accounting reports
Processing hardware, 3, 5–6; *see also* Hardware

Processing unit, 3
Processor, 5
Program, 2
Prosthetic devices, 156, 162–64; *see also* Assistive devices
Protocols, 9
PubMed, 10, 187, 190; *see also* Medical literature databases
Puff straws, 160; *see also* Assistive devices
Pulmonary monitors, 157

R

Radiology, 79–89
   digital imaging techniques, 82–86
   ultrasound, 81
   X-rays, 80–81
Random access memory (RAM), 6; *see also* Memory
Rational drug design, 134–35
Read only memory (ROM), 6; *see also* Memory
Records, 44
Relational database, 43
Reliability of health information on the Internet, 194–95
Remineralize, 108
Remote monitoring devices, 65; *see also* Telehome care
Resource utilization groups (RUGs), 51
Restricting access, biometric methods, 24–25; *see also* Security
   biometric keyboards, 24
   body odor sensors, 24
   facial structure scans, 25
   facial thermography, 24
   fingerprints, 24
   hand prints, 24
   iris scans, 24
   lip prints, 24
   retina scans, 24
Retina scans, 24; *see also* Biometric methods of restricting access
Right to Financial Privacy Act of 1978, 23
Risks posed by implants, 166
RNA interference (RNAi), 137
ROBODOC, 119; *see also* Computer-assisted surgery
Robotics, computer-assisted surgery and, 118–22

Robots, 116–22, 140–42
  in hospital pharmacies, 142
  in pharmacies, 140–41
  in surgery, 116–22
RNAi. *see* RNA interference
RUGs. *see* Resource utilization groups

S

Scanning devices, 4; *see also* Input devices
Schedule of benefits, 47
Scientific visualization, 83, 135
Screen reader software, 159
SDILINE (Selective Dissemination of
      Information Online), 187; *see also*
      Medical literature databases
Search engine, 10
Secondary storage devices, 3, 6; *see also*
      Hardware
Secondary storage media, 6
  magnetic disk, 6
  magnetic tape, 6
  optical disk, 6
    compact disk (CD), 6
    digital video disk (DVD), 6
Security, 22–25, 29–33
  codes of conduct, 22
  encryption, 22
  and health care, 29–33
  overview of, 20–21
  methods of restricting access, 22–25
    firewalls, 25
    passwords, 24
    PINs, 24
    biometric methods of restricting
      access, 24–25
Self-help, 192–93, 195
  software, 195
  on the Web, 192–93; *see also* Internet
Silicon chip, 3
Simulation, 178–81; *see also* Education
  software, 178
  virtual reality, 178–81
Simulators, human patient, 181–84
Social implications, 211
Social Security Online Privacy Protection
      Act of 2001, 24
SOCRATES, 123; *see also* Computer-
      assisted surgery

Soft copy, 6
Software, 6–8
  administrative, 44–46
  application, 7–8
  communications, 8
  database management systems
    (DBMS), 7
  electronic spreadsheets, 7
  graphics, 7
  MediSoft, 7, 43, 50
  screen reader, 159
  self-help, 195
  simulation, 178
  system, 7
  word processing, 7
Software piracy, 21
Speaker-independent/dependent speech
    recognition systems, 159
Specialization in dentistry, growth of,
    109; *see also* Dentistry
Special purpose applications, 42; *see also*
    Applications
  future trends, 208–10
SPECT (single photon emission computed
    tomography), 82; *see also* Digital
    imaging techniques
Speech recognition systems, 159–60;*see*
    also Assistive devices
Speech synthesizers, 159
Spreadsheets, electronic, 7; *see also* Software
Starbright World, 193
Stereotactic radiosurgery, 86–87; *see also*
    Bloodless surgery
Store-and-forward technology, 61
Superbill, 46, 50; *see also* Encounter form
Support groups on the Web, 193; *see also*
    Internet
Surgery, 115–27
  bloodless, 80, 86–87
  computer-assisted, 116–26
  in dentistry, 109
  lasers in, 124
  telepresence (distance), 123
System board, 5
System software, 7; *see also* Software
System unit, 5

T

Tables, 44

TCP/IP (transmission control protocol/Internet protocol), 10
Telecardiology, 63
Telecommunications, 8–9; *see also* Communication
  overview of, 8–9
  uses of, 9
Telecommunications Act of 1996, 68, 69
Telecommunications networks, 8
Teleconferencing, 61, 62, 64, 66; *see also* Interactive videoconferencing
Teledentistry, 109
Teledermatology, 62
Telehome care, 60, 65–66
  remote monitoring devices, 65
Telemedicine, 42, 59–70
  issues in, 68–70
  overview of, 60–61
  in prison, 66–67
  privacy and, 32
  uses of, 67–68
Telenursing, 68
Teleoncology, 60
Telepathology, 62
Telepharmacy, 143–45
Telepresence (distance) surgery, 116, 123; *see also* Computer-assisted surgery
Telepsychiatry, 60, 64–65
Teleradiology, 61–62
Telespirometry, 65; *see also* Remote monitoring devices
Telestroke, 63–64
Teletriage, 68
Text telephones, 160; *see also* Assistive devices
Theft of information, 21
Theft of services, 21
Tonometers, 158
Topography, corneal, 158
Total Information Awareness Program, 28
Tracey Visual Function Analyzer, 158
Transactions, 46
TRICARE, 47

U

Ultrafast CT, 82–83

Ultrasound, 81
URL (uniform resource locator), 10
USA Patriot Act of 2001, 23, 27–28
  privacy of medical records under, 31–32
User interface, 7

V

Videoconferencing. *see* Interactive video-conferencing
Video Privacy Protection Act (1988), 23
Video Voyeurism Act of 2001, 24
Virtual environment, 116
Virtual Hospital, 185
Virtual human embryo, 177
Virtual reality simulations, 178–81; *see also* Education
  epidural simulator, 180
  KISMET, 178
  patient simulators, 18, 182, 183, 184
Virtual reality (VR), 116
Viruses, computer, 20
Visible Human Project, 176–77

W

Web. *see* World Wide Web (WWW)
Web browser, 10
Web sites, 10
Wide area networks (WANs), 8
Word processing, 7
Workers' compensation, 48
World Wide Web (WWW), 2, 9–11; *see also* Internet

X

X-rays, 80–81, 104; *see also* Diagnostic tools

Z

ZEUS, 120; *see also* Surgery